ASTANGA YOGA FOR YOU

The Comprehensive Guide to Power Yoga at Home for Everyone

TARA FRASER

DUNCAN BAIRD PUBLISHERS

LONDON

For Nigel

Astanga Yoga for You
Tara Fraser

This revised edition first published in the United Kingdom and Ireland in 2007 by
Duncan Baird Publishers Ltd
Sixth Floor, Castle House
75-76 Wells Street
London W1T 3QH

Created and designed by Duncan Baird Publishers
Copyright © Duncan Baird Publishers 2005, 2007
Text copyright © Tara Fraser 2005, 2007
Commissioned photography copyright © Duncan Baird Publishers 2005

Managing Editor: Julia Charles
Editor: Kesta Desmond
Managing Designer: Dan Sturges
Designers: Suzanne Tuhrim, Allan Sommerville
Picture Researcher: Julia Ruxton
Commissioned photography: Matthew Ward
Commissioned artwork: Debbie Maizels

British Library Cataloguing-in-Publication Data:
A catalogue record for this book is available from the British Library

10 9 8 7 6 5 4 3 2 1

ISBN: 978-1-84483-366-5

Typeset in GillSans and Joanna MT
Colour reproduction by Scanhouse, Malaysia
Printed in Singapore by Imago

Note on abbreviations:
BCE (Before the Common Era) is the equivalent of BC.
CE (Common Era) is the equivalent of AD.

Publisher's note:
Before following any advice or practice suggested in this book, it is recommended that you
consult your doctor as to its suitability, especially if you suffer from any health problems or
special conditions. The publishers, the author and the photographers cannot accept responsibility
for any injuries or damage incurred as a result of following the exercises in this book, or of using
any of the therapeutic methods described or mentioned here.

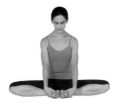

"You cannot teach a man anything;
you can only help him find it within himself."
Galileo Galilei

contents

introduction

When I was asked to write this book I found myself in a bit of a dilemma. I love yoga and had dabbled with Astanga yoga for years, enjoying its powerful, fluid style. I was excited by the prospect of researching and observing this unique form of Hatha yoga, but I also wondered whether it would be possible for me to undertake such a task. For a start, I found many of the postures difficult and I had to be willing to be photographed attempting all of them!

As I could not claim to be an "expert" in Astanga yoga, this book has been a research project for me. I have tried to make a worthwhile contribution from an outsider's perspective. Drawing on the experience and advice of Astanga teachers and practitioners as well as my own experiences learning, practising and teaching, I pieced together a clearer picture. I have approached the subject as an explorer and a beginner rather than a devotee. Wherever possible I have asked questions and challenged assumptions. I have used my knowledge and expertise in other forms of yoga to try to apply a critical eye to this form, to describe its essential characteristics and analyze what has made it so popular.

I have included in the book some of the answers to the many questions that arose in my research. I have felt inspired, frustrated, elated and distraught by this practice, and I am hugely grateful to everyone who coaxed, pushed, pulled and carried me through the process of getting my experiences down on paper. I humbly offer this book as a guide to beginners and tentative dabblers, with the hope that it inspires you to take the plunge. There is nothing quite like Astanga yoga; it is glorious, captivating, astonishing and, most importantly, for you!

Tara Fraser

how to use this book

This book is a reference manual for Astanga yoga. I do not recommend that you learn Astanga yoga solely from a book – its very nature makes this almost impossible and potentially risky. If you are familiar with another form of yoga, this book may be useful in starting off an Astanga yoga practice and comparing it to the style you know. If you are a total novice, there is enough basic information here to help you decide if this kind of yoga is for you – if it isn't, try looking at my book *Yoga for You* which contains a range of gentle practices, safe to do by yourself at home. In all cases, you will need to find a good teacher, and thanks to the huge popularity of this form of yoga, this is getting easier to do.

Use this book to supplement the classes you attend. It will help you to remember the key aspects and the order of the postures. I have included information about the history, theory and principles of the practice (chapters 1–3) and in Chapter 4 you will find find Astanga yoga postures in sequence with their suggested modifications. Please read at least chapters 3 and 4 before leaping to your mat to start a practice! Chapter 5 offers a few ideas and resources for deepening or broadening your understanding of yoga in general and Astanga yoga specifically. I have included book titles for further reading, but remember: "99 percent practice, one percent theory!"

SYMBOLS USED IN THIS BOOK

An easier modification of a posture to be used if you are a beginner, if you are having difficulty in a pose or if you simply want a softer yoga practice.

Ideas, tips and comments that will help you in a posture.

Drishti (gazing point; see page 39).

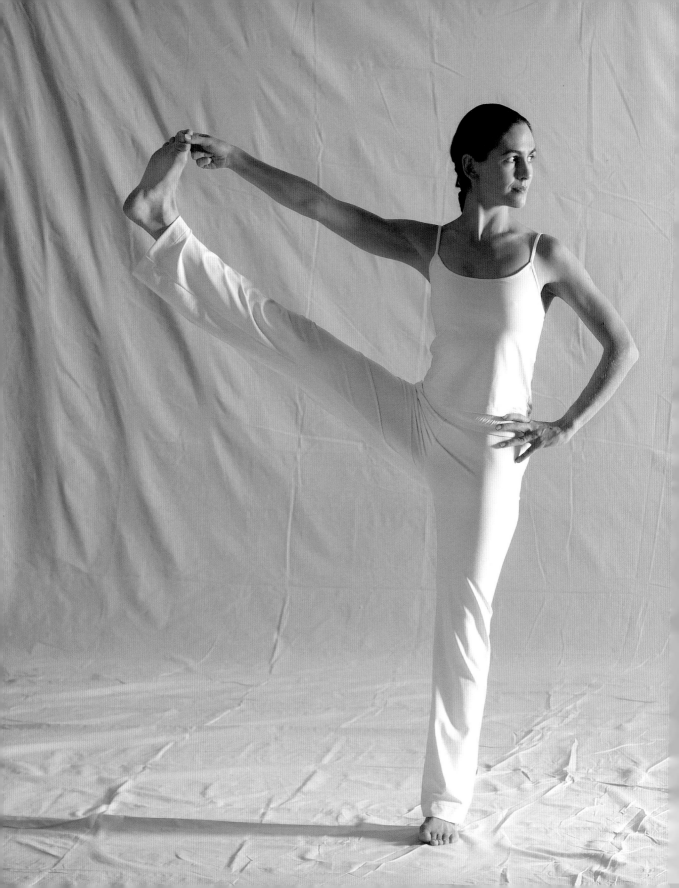

chapter one

the roots of a tradition

Astanga Vinyasa yoga has had an extraordinary impact on the
modern western world. People from all walks of life – from
film stars to city stockbrokers – are now swearing by its
magical properties. Yoga books and magazines often proclaim
the benefits of this "2,000-year-old practice" from India. But
exactly how old is the practice of Astanga Vinyasa yoga and
what do we know about the men who brought it to the
wider world, and specifically to its mass popularity in the
modern West? Why is it that such a strenuous and demanding
practice requiring huge self-discipline has proved to be
so popular in a culture better known for its increasingly
sedentary and consumer-orientated lifestyles?

the history of astanga yoga

The history of yoga is complex and elusive. It covers a vast time-span, a huge area and is largely uncatalogued. Although texts relating to yoga exist, many may have been lost or destroyed. Untangling the precise history of yoga is almost impossible – something which helps to preserve yoga's mystique.

Yoga is part of a system of Indian philosophy which appeared around 2,000 years ago. Its key text, *Yoga Sutras of Patanjali* (see pages 18–19), is primarily concerned with the nature of the mind. It does not include descriptions of yoga postures, mentioning only a seated pose for meditation. The form of yoga that works through the medium of the physical body using postures, breathing exercises and cleansing practices is known as Hatha yoga, and it is derived from a number of different traditions including classical yoga and Tantric texts. The aim of Hatha yoga is liberation from the cycle of rebirth within one lifetime (the term "Hatha" means "forceful"). Practising yoga can also take the form of worship (Bhakti yoga), performing selfless acts of work (Karma yoga) or acquiring knowledge (Jnana yoga).

Hatha yoga has been practised in various forms for many hundreds of years. Within Hatha yoga are various branches or styles of yoga of which Astanga Vinyasa is one.

Yoga Kurunta

The core practice of Astanga Vinyasa is a set sequence of postures (*asanas*) that is said to have been described in a text called the *Yoga Kurunta*. True to form, very little is known about this legendary text; it cannot accurately be dated (although it may be up to 1,000 years old), and its author,

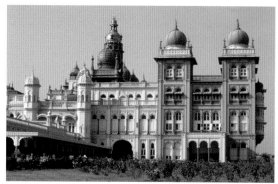

Mysore Palace in India is a key place in the history of Astanga yoga. This is where, from 1933–1955, Professor Krishnamacharya taught the techniques of Astanga yoga reputedly derived from the *Yoga Kurunta*.

a *rishi* (seer) named Vamana, was either the compiler of the method of Astanga yoga or possibly its inventor. We know about the *Yoga Kurunta* because Professor Krishnamacharya (see pages 16–17), one of the modern world's most revered yogis, said that he was taught the contents of all or part of the *Yoga Kurunta* by his teacher Shri Ramamohan Brahmachari in the Himalayas in the 1920s. He is also said to have studied a copy of the text in a library in Calcutta in the early 1930s. Unfortunately, this copy was reputedly eaten by ants, and no other copy is known to exist. Somewhat confusingly, another branch of Hatha yoga – Iyengar yoga – also uses the term "yoga *korunta*" but in this case it refers to the use of ropes in yoga practice.

The characteristics of Astanga Vinyasa

The *Yoga Kurunta* is said to have described three series of postures: *Yoga Chikitsa* (yoga therapy) which we know as the "Primary Series"; *Nadi Sodhana* (channel cleansing) known as the "Intermediate series"; and *Sthira Bhaga* (divine stability) which can be broken down into four parts and is known as the "Advanced Series". Postures within each series are connected by specific movements that act as counterposes, known as "vinyasa". These three series probably represent the most physically challenging type of yoga practice ever constructed. This book only shows the postures of the

Primary Series, which are principally forward bends of various kinds. The Intermediate Series contains a lot of back-bending poses and the Advanced Series contains more variations of both with some difficult balances.

Apart from the use of vinyasa, other key characteristics of Astanga yoga detailed in the *Yoga Kurunta* are the continuous use of techniques known as *ujjayi* breathing (see page 36) and *bandhas* (see pages 35–37) throughout a yoga practice. Practitioners become very hot which facilitates purificatory sweating and enables deep stretching without injury.

Astanga yoga in the West

Astanga yoga started to spread to America in the 1970s when students studied in India with Shri K Pattabhi Jois (see pages 14–15) and returned home to teach his techniques to others. Many of these early students continue to study with Shri K Pattabhi Jois and have been teaching his method for decades. Some have stuck fairly strictly to the system as it was introduced to them. Others have developed variations based on their own experience, and this has led to a flowering of diverse styles that are known as "vinyasa-based". These types of Hatha yoga maintain the fluid movement, style and breathing pattern of Astanga Vinyasa yoga but have included postures other than those taught by Shri K Pattabhi Jois in the original form.

It is difficult to say exactly why Astanga yoga appeals to people from all walks of life all over the world. Perhaps there is something reassuring about following a strict regime in a life that has become bewilderingly full of choices.

Professor Krishnamacharya often toured with groups of students performing yoga to interest people in the practice. Here, he is seen demonstrating with his students in the courtyard of Mysore Palace.

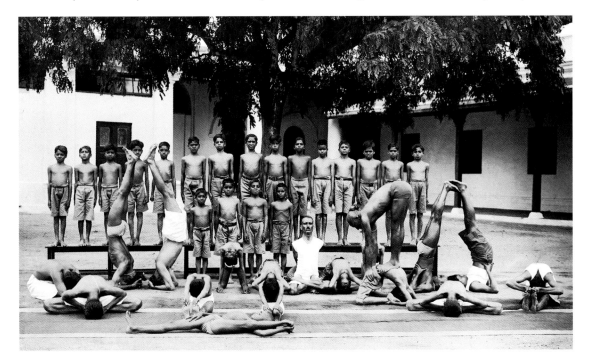

shri k pattabhi jois

Shri K Pattabhi Jois is the modern guru of Astanga yoga. Beloved by his students the world over, he is affectionately known by them as "Guruji". He gained his reputation not by talking about yoga or having a flamboyant personality, but by emphasizing his doctrine of "99 percent practice, one percent theory". He teaches simply, giving powerful hands-on adjustments to students and talking them through the series of postures that he has dedicated his life to studying, practising and teaching.

Early life

Shri K Pattabhi Jois was born in July 1915, the fifth in a family of nine children of the Brahmin caste (the priestly caste in Hinduism). The family lived in a small village in a district of Mysore in South India. His father was an astrologer and priest with no recorded interest in yoga – yoga was regarded somewhat suspiciously by many Brahmin families as an esoteric practice unsuitable for a family man or a young Brahmin boy. So, Pattabhi Jois didn't tell his parents when he went to see a yoga lecture and demonstration at his local hall in November 1927. He was 12-years-old and had little idea of what the lecture was about, but the demonstration made a huge impression upon him. The yogi had a powerful and athletic physique, and appeared to float through the air, land as delicately as a cat and perform amazing feats of breath control. Pattabhi Jois resolved to ask this man to take him on as a student. He was accepted and began his study with Professor Krishnamacharya (see pages 16–17).

Studying with Krishnamacharya

Every morning Pattabhi Jois studied *asana* (postures) with Krishnamacharya before going to school. He learned the postures very quickly because he was young and fit. After two years he stopped studying yoga with Krishnamacharya when he went to the Sanskrit College in Mysore and they lost contact with one another. By chance their paths crossed again in 1931 when Pattabhi Jois attended another yoga demonstration given by Krishnamacharya in Mysore. Having re-established contact, he resumed his study of yoga and continued for the next two decades. After mastering *asana*, he

was taught *pranayama* (breathing techniques) and meditation. Pattabhi Jois has described Krishnamacharya as a strict and strong teacher, who demanded high standards and punished minute transgressions. But he also talks about his teacher with great affection.

In March 1937 the Maharaja of Mysore appointed Pattabhi Jois as the Head of Yoga at the Sanskrit College, despite the fact that he was still studying as a student there. In 1956 he was promoted to Professor of Sanskrit and Advaita Vedanta. He continued to work at the college until his retirement in 1973.

Family life

Shri K Pattabhi Jois married Savitramma, the daughter of a Sanskrit scholar called Narayana Shastria, in June 1937. He was 22-years-old and she was 14. Known simply as Amma (mother), she was his student and reputedly learned all of the series of Astanga yoga from Pattabhi Jois and was awarded a teaching certificate from Krishnamacharya. Life was hard at the beginning; they didn't have a lot of money to live on and they soon had three children – Saraswati, Manju and Ramesh – to support. In the photographs of Amma and Guruji celebrating his 80th birthday in 1995 she is smiling, confident and affectionate (although she is said to have been quite in awe of Pattabhi Jois in the early part of their marriage). At Amma's death in 1997, Pattabhi Jois initiated a series of projects to renovate and build new temples in his home village of Kowshika in her memory. Saraswati, their daughter, had a son, Sharath Rangaswamy in 1971, who is currently co-director of the yoga school in Mysore.

Born in 1915, Shri K Pattabhi Jois or "Guruji" is the contemporary guru of Astanga yoga. He has taught the techniques of Astanga yoga to students all over the world.

The Astanga Yoga Research Institute

In 1948 Shri K Pattabhi Jois' students helped him to buy a home in Laxmipuram where he established The Astanga Yoga Research Institute. This grand title belied the small and very modest building in which the Institute was housed. The Institute was to provide space for Pattabhi Jois to teach his students, and a base from which to research the curative and health benefits of yoga.

By 1964 the number of students was growing steadily and the Institute was extended to provide a bigger yoga space and a resting room. The first Westerner to study with Pattabhi Jois around this time was Andre van Lysebeth who spent two months learning Astanga yoga. Van Lysebeth later wrote a book called *Pranayama* in which he listed Pattabhi Jois' name and address. This marked the beginning of a trickle of Western students to Mysore; it soon turned into a stream, and is now a full blown river with thousands of students ranging from curious beginners to seasoned and faithful devotees turning up to study yoga. Curiously, the vast majority of students are from the West with very few Indians taking an interest in Astanga yoga.

Yoga Mala

In 1958, Pattabhi Jois began work on *Yoga Mala*, the book that gives detailed instructions for all of the postures that he was then teaching in the Primary Series, plus background information on the methodology and theory of yoga practice. *Yoga Mala* was published in the Kanada language in 1962; an English translation appeared in 1999. Pattabhi Jois mentions the text from which Astanga yoga is said to originate, the *Yoga Kurunta* (see page 12); although he has said that he never saw the text himself, he believed that Krishnamacharya had seen it and had taught him the ancient system of Astanga yoga faithfully from the *Yoga Kurunta*.

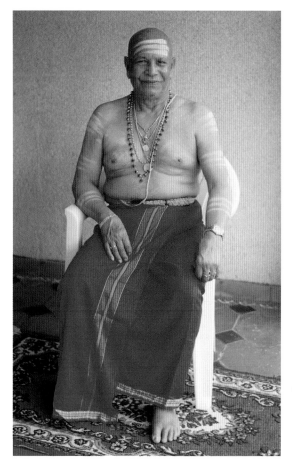

Shri K Pattabhi Jois today

For some years in the early 1970s, Pattabhi Jois taught yoga as a therapeutic method at the Ayurvedic College in Mysore. In 1975 he was invited to the US to teach a handful of students in California – the beginning of the arrival of Astanga yoga in the West. Today he tours the world assisted by his grandson Sharath and teaches at home in his yoga *shala* (school). Even at his advanced age Pattabhi Jois has great stamina and strength, kind eyes and a warm smile. He is a living advertisement for the positive powers of yoga.

professor krishnamacharya

Born on the 18th November 1888 in Mysore, India, Tirumalai Krishnamacharya was to become the most influential yoga teacher in the modern world. His emphasis on the curative and transformational potential of *asana* practice has become the mainstay of modern yoga.

Studying yoga

Krishnamacharya began his study of Sanskrit and yoga with his father at the age of five. Later, he took Sanskrit, logic and grammar at Banaras University where he was well known for his outstanding academic capabilities. While studying he heard of a great yogi, Shri Ramamohan Brahmachari, who lived near Lake Manasarovar in Tibet. It became Krishnamacharya's deepest wish to study with this man and so in 1916 he undertook the perilous journey north toward Mount Kailash in the Himalayas. After considerable persuasion (as is traditional) Shri Ramamohan Brahmachari took on Krishnamacharya as his student. Over a period of seven years, Krishnamacharya is reputed to have learned more than 3,000 *asanas*, *pranayama* and studied texts including the *Yoga Sutras of Patanjali* (see pages 18–19) and the *Yoga Kurunta* (see page 12).

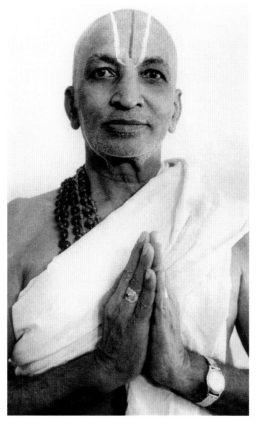

Krishnamacharya devoted his life to studying yoga, philosophy, Ayurveda, grammar, astrology, music and religion. He is described as an outspoken man with a towering intellect.

Spreading the message

On leaving, Shri Ramamohan Brahmachari told Krishnamacharya to live a family life but also to use his tal-ents to spread the message of yoga and to help to heal the sick. So, forgoing a career in academia that would have rewarded him handsomely, he returned to the south of India to study Ayurveda and to teach yoga, a job that was poorly paid and not well respected. He studied texts written in his native Tamil and combined these with the teachings he had learned from Shri Ramamohan Brahmachari, giving him a uniquely broad sphere of knowledge.

The yoga *shala* at Mysore Palace

In 1924 Krishnamacharya returned to his home district of Mysore, and from 1933–1955 taught yoga at the Mysore Palace with the encouragement of the Maharajah (prince) of Mysore, Krishnarajendra Woodyar IV, who was devoted to yoga. Krishnamacharya wrote his first book, *Yoga Makarandam* ("Secrets of Yoga"), here and seemed to flourish in the Palace environment. The Palace gymnasium became his yoga *shala* (school). Contemporary photographs show a high ceilinged room with a vaulting-horse, ropes, wall bars and what look like early rowing machines and crash mats. Krishnamacharya himself was an impressive looking athlete.

Krishnamacharya's yoga *shala* at the Palace eventually had to close, partly because the Maharaja died in 1940 – and his son did not share his devotion to yoga – and partly because of Professor Krishnamacharya's reputation for being a teacher who was tough on his students.

Krishnamacharya's students

Although he never travelled to the West himself, Professor Krishnamacharya's students have exported his teaching with great success. The four students who have been most instrumental in bringing yoga to the West are Shri K Pattabhi Jois (see pages 14–15), Indra Devi, BKS Iyengar and TKV Desikachar (Krishnamacharya's son).

Indra Devi (a Latvian whose original name was Zhenia Labunskaia) came to study with Krishnamacharya in 1937. He turned her away at first (being both a woman and a Westerner). Eventually, when she rose to every challenge he set, he took her on as his pupil. This was a powerful decision for a devout Brahmin to make – it went against tradition and threatened his own reputation and standing. Subsequently Krishnamacharya did much to promote the study of yoga for women and girls, and all of his own children did yoga.

BKS Iyengar – who later became his brother-in-law, studied with Krishnamacharya for about a year. He has always shown deep respect for his teacher, and dedicated his seminal text *Light on Yoga* to him, yet he described his training as harsh and his teacher as "intellectually intoxicated".

So many great figures in history present a hard act to follow, yet Krishnamacharya's students have continued to develop his teaching in very different ways, while maintaining the deepest respect for their guru and his methods.

Later life

Finally, Krishnamacharya settled with his family in Madras where he continued to teach. He had six children of whom two, Shri Bashyam and TKV Desikachar, have continued to teach yoga. TKV Desikachar studied yoga with his father towards the end of Krishnamacharya's life. In 1976 TKV Desikachar founded the Krishnamacharya Yoga *Mandiram* as a place in which to carry on the work of his father; it exists to this day as a thriving centre for the study of yoga.

Krishnamacharya's later teaching, in contrast to the early work based on the strict system of Astanga yoga, emphasized the individual nature of a yoga practice and of healing; no two people are the same. He used pulse diagnosis and Ayurvedic skills to help diagnose and prescribe specific yoga practice, diet and lifestyle changes for his students. Throughout his life the *Yoga Sutras of Patanjali* was the most important text to Krishnamacharya, but he also drew upon his vast knowledge of other systems in his teaching, including a text known as the *Yoga Rahasya* and Ayurvedic treatise. With a formidable constitution and boundless energy Krishnamacharya continued teaching until just six weeks before his death in 1989.

Krishnamacharya's legacy

The full extent of Krishnamacharya's legacy remains to be revealed. His techniques have become the "standard" methods of yoga in many cases. The combining of breath and posture work to create a moving meditation, the development of carefully ordered practice emphasizing the curative quality of *asana* and the emphasis on inverted postures (head- and shoulderstands) stem principally from the work of Krishnamacharya.

It is difficult to say how much of the material that Krishnamacharya taught was derived from the teaching he had received from Ramamohan and the *Yoga Kurunta*, and how much was his own synthesis or invention. Certainly, in his lifetime he never claimed credit for any of the work he did, always referring back to his own teacher or a more ancient source. However, he was clearly a great innovator and it seems likely that much of the material he developed could be attributed directly to him – even if his inspiration lay with a higher power.

patanjali's eight-limbed path

The term Astanga yoga means "eight-limbed yoga" and it comes from an aphorism in a roughly 2,000-year-old Sanskrit text known as the *Yoga Sutras of Patanjali* – the cornerstone of classical yoga philosophy. Posture and breath control – the two fundamental practices of Astanga yoga – are described as the third and fourth limbs in Patanjali's eight-limbed path to self-realization.

Sutras on a range of subjects abound in Indian culture. The word *sutra* means literally "a thread" and is used to denote a particular form of written and oral communication. The deliberately dense and compact form of the *sutras* suits their purpose exactly: the short, pithy statements are easy to memorize and chant, and they can be passed on from guru to student with great accuracy without the need for textbooks. Because of the terse style in which the *sutras* are written, students of yoga must rely on a guru to interpret, unravel and expound the philosophy contained within each one. The meaning of each *sutra* may also be tailored to a student's individual needs. This keeps alive both the oral tradition and the guru-student relationship.

Patanjali's text consists of 195 *sutras* that are presented in four chapters. The first chapter describes the path of yoga and includes right at the beginning the classical definition of yoga: *yoga citta vrtti nirodha* ("yoga is the ability to control the fluctuations of the mind"). The "eight limbs" are described in Chapter Two, whose title – *sadhanapada* – can be interpreted as "method". In Chapter Two, *Sutra* 2:29 lists the eight principles by which, when unaffected by adverse circumstances, we should live:

1. **Yama**: social conduct. This includes *ahimsa* (non-violence), *satya* (truthfulness), *asteya* (non-stealing), *brahmacarya* (moderation in sex and in all things) and *aparigraha* (non-greed).
2. **Niyama**: individual conduct. This includes: *sauca* (purity or cleanliness), *santosa* (contentment), *tapas* (austerity), *svadhyaya* (the study of texts), *isvarapranidhana* (awareness of and devotion to the highest – the "highest" doesn't have to be a religious concept; it is open to individual definition).
3. **Asana**: posture, which should be stable (*sthira*) and open (*sukha*) for meditation.
4. **Pranayama**: breath control which should be refined to help concentrate one's thoughts.
5. **Pratyahara**: sense withdrawal to enhance inner perception.
6. **Dharana**: concentration; focusing on a particular point.
7. **Dhyana**: meditation, a state that arises when concentration is refined.

WHO WAS PATANJALI?

Although the *Yoga Sutras of Patanjali* is one of the most important ancient texts on yoga, its author remains enigmatic – very little is known about his life. Patanjali is generally thought to have been the "compiler" of the text rather than its originator. This is because the teachings appear to be part of a much older oral tradition. Indeed scholars argue about the construction of the text, for example, whether one or more of its four chapters are later additions, whether different schools of thought are conflated into a single text, and so on.

The name Patanjali can be broken into two parts: "Pat" meaning "to fall", and "anjali", a gesture of giving and receiving. So perhaps Patanjali is an appropriate name chosen for the compiler of a philosophy that fell as a gift into the open hands of mankind.

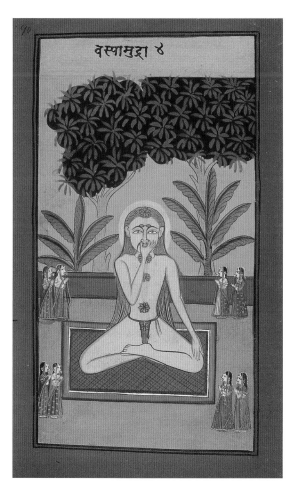

वस्त्रामुद्रा ४

This Indian miniature painting from the 18th century BCE shows a yogi practising *pranayama* (breath control), the fourth limb of yoga.

8. **Samadhi**: the superconscious state; self-realization; cognitive unification. The state of *samadhi* develops in stages and has "side effects" – supernatural powers (*siddhis*). Its ultimate point is total freedom from all the ties of existence.

The eight limbs in practice

According to Patanjali's text, following the eight limbs enables a diligent student to obtain the clarity of perception necessary to achieve enlightenment or self-realization.

Shri K Patthabi Jois (see pages 14–15) describes the first four limbs as "external" and the last four as "internal". Although he regards the practice of yoga *asana* as the primary basis for all other work he puts great emphasis on the order of the limbs, saying that it is impossible to go back to correct mistakes later if you progress without care. Each limb (and each posture of his series) must be perfected before the next is attempted.

The order of practice of the eight limbs is a subject of debate in the yoga world. It is difficult to say whether it is indeed essential to have grasped limbs one and two (*yama* and *niyama*) before starting the practice of *asana*. A literal translation of the text seems to indicate that the steps must be performed in strict sequence. Others argue that various limbs can be worked on simultaneously. In reality, many of us start with the practice of postures, which leads us to a greater awareness of our breath, and eventually an improved control of breath and concentration. It seems that greater awareness on this physical level can and often does lead yoga students to examine their social and personal conduct. After a period of study, many individuals go on to make radical changes in their lives.

To a large extent, the practice of Astanga yoga encompasses the "internal limbs" of Patanjali's *sutras*. The intense concentration required to perform the Primary Series results in a kind of meditation in movement. Eventually, it is possible to experience a quality of total absorption that may be related to lower levels of the state of *samadhi*. Even if you don't specifically set out to explore the internal limbs in your Astanga yoga practice, you may find that they happen naturally. The principles of sense withdrawal, concentration, meditation and self-realization, once seeded in your mind, have a way of expressing themselves at a time when you are sufficiently open to receive and act upon them.

astanga yoga in the modern world

There has been a yoga boom in the West. It started in America and has spread across the whole of the developed world and even back to India, where it was still considered a rather fringe activity until relatively recently. In the US, a poll commissioned by *Yoga Journal* found that more than six million Americans practise yoga and close to 17 million more expressed an interest in yoga.

Times have changed since Astanga yoga first evolved. Modern Westerners live very different lives from those of Krishnamacharya and his contemporaries. Part of the appeal of yoga for many is that it originates from a "simpler" time, when life was less pressured and more in tune with nature. As such, yoga is often perceived as a short-cut to a more holistic, balanced lifestyle. The danger in this is that, unless we make a fundamental shift in lifestyle, adding yoga to an already hectic schedule can simply serve to increase our overall stress levels and sense of performance pressure. It is not the same to practise yoga in monastic seclusion as it is to combine it with a full-time job, family and social life.

The popularity of Astanga yoga

Astanga yoga has become one of the more fashionable styles of yoga in the West and there are several reasons for this. Many high-profile celebrities practise Astanga and it is popularly perceived as a way to develop a beautiful, toned and muscular physique. The highly acrobatic and aesthetic appearance of the postures themselves are also appealing and impressive to many people.

In recent years yoga has been commercialized to the extent that it is now possible to buy designer yoga outfits and go on five-star luxury yoga holidays. Astanga yoga may

The increasing popularity of Astanga yoga means that many people incorporate their yoga practice into an already busy schedule of activities.

also be appealing to our competitive spirit – it is very easy to compare your practice to another person's or see Astanga yoga as another aspirational lifestyle goal, like a better suntan or a faster car. In a more positive sense, the strict methods and sequence of postures of Astanga yoga may also account for its popularity – in a culture in which we are overwhelmed by variety Astanga yoga provides a welcome respite. Traditionally, you just do it – you don't ask questions!

The benefits and the drawbacks

Astanga yoga is a remarkable tool for enabling calm; it is an oasis in a hectic world. For those devoted to this practice it provides a way to free the body of pent-up tensions and release the mind from stress – ultimately, it is a good way to know your limits and develop the strengths you need to cope in a modern urban environment.

The benefits of being an Astanga yoga practitioner are undoubted, but it is important to know that this style of yoga is a powerful tool that can have profound physical and emotional effects. If you are doing it on top of your regular lifestyle rather than instead of it, you may well get some unwelcome side effects (see page 25). This is not a reason to give up the practice, but some adjustment may be necessary. If you are already rushed off your feet and feeling stressed,

Astanga yoga may be a struggle to maintain and it may be worth trying a reduced practice (for example, the short practice on pages 120–121). Alternatively, you can consider changing your lifestyle.

Astanga yoga stokes up a terrific amount of energy, you need to be able to channel this properly in your daily life or it can get out of hand. Energy should be used for positive things in your life, whatever they may be, however simple or small. The traditional warnings to lead a *sattvic* (pure) life are not out of place even, or perhaps especially, in our modern setting. You need to eat and sleep well, and avoid the use of drugs and stimulants. Dietary and lifestyle changes need to take place gradually, and for most people they are spontaneous – the more yoga you do, the more aware you are of your body's reaction to foods, drugs and chemicals.

The spirit of Astanga yoga

The yoga boom has been facilitated by the introduction of Astanga (and other styles of yoga) classes into health clubs and gyms of every major city in the West, and now even in smaller towns and rural places too. Some people fear that this has resulted in the dumbing down of Astanga yoga, turning it into a physical workout and detaching it from its noble origins as a spiritual practice. While this is a valid fear, it should be noted that among Krishnamacharya's probable influences in his early teaching was the training regimes of Indian gymnasts and wrestlers. Krishnamacharya himself was very likely the innovator of many of the aspects of Astanga yoga that we now consider "traditional". As befits a living, breathing tradition we should be seeking to improve and refine what we do at all times. The world of sports, gymnastics and dance have many positive skills and qualities that can be usefully integrated into a yoga practice, and cross-fertilization between these forms need not necessarily be seen as a bad thing. Yoga is a state of mind rather than a strict series of actions and this can be applied to any task you do, whether it is dishwashing, running a marathon or doing the Primary Series.

VARIATIONS ON ASTANGA YOGA

Some teachers feel that it is important to adhere strictly to the set sequence of postures that make up the Primary Series. Others view Astanga yoga as a living tradition that varies in its detail from one teacher to the next. For example, different Western teachers who have studied with Shri K Pattabhi Jois at different times have returned with small variations on the sequence. In addition, some teachers have heavily modified the sequence to create their own style – maintaining the principles of heat, *bandha* and vinyasa but selecting very different *asana*. Many of these forms are more accessible to average students than the traditional Astanga Vinyasa sequences.

Astanga yoga was found by some students and teachers to be limited and hard to perfect in its strict form, and this has led to the creation of classes based on Astanga yoga that are described as Dynamic Yoga or Vinyasa Flow. Although this can be seen as a corruption of the form, on the positive side it has introduced thousands of people to yoga who might otherwise never have come across it.

Learning in a gym environment

Teaching quality in health clubs and gyms ranges from the frankly deplorable to world class excellence. Because yoga teaching is largely unregulated, you need to rely on intuition and common sense when choosing a class. In gym environments, the competitive aspects of sport may be heavily emphasized. It may be almost impossible to avoid being sucked into a competitive frame of mind – something that is counter to the yoga philosophy. You also risk injury if you try to force your body into a pose. If you are learning yoga in a gym environment, take care to keep your yoga personal and balanced – above all don't compete with your classmates.

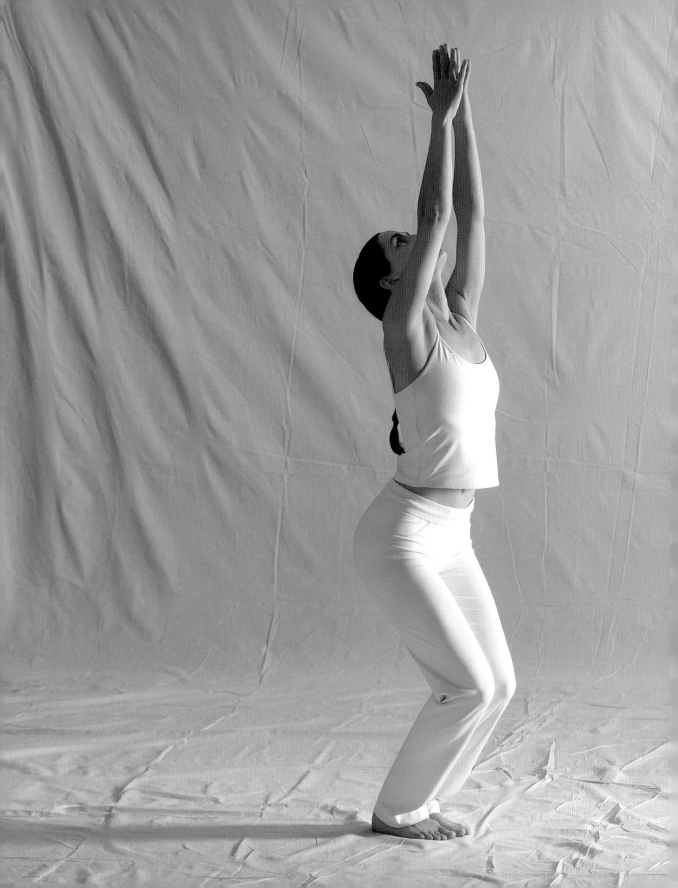

creating a personal practice

One of the unique qualities of Astanga yoga is that it provides a yardstick with which to measure our lives and our deeper selves. Because we do the same practice each time, we develop an acute awareness of anything that differs in the way we feel or behave. We can use the practice as a way of being in touch with our inner selves from day to day and year to year. But to fully appreciate the benefits of such a practice and to be able to sustain it for years, we need to approach Astanga yoga with care and acknowledge its terrific power. This chapter examines the origins and intentions of the teachings of Astanga yoga, and how you can turn them to your advantage in the highly pressurized environments in which many of us live.

the benefits of astanga yoga

Taking up yoga can radically change your outlook, the way you feel and the way that you choose to live your life. Astanga yoga is a particularly intense and disciplined form of practice and, although you will begin to feel many beneficial changes right from the start, others will take months or years to become apparent.

The physical benefits

The early benefits of Astanga yoga practice include improved balance and co-ordination, and feeling more healthy, alert, vibrant and energetic. The constant repetition of a wide range of postures quickly improves your levels of fitness. You develop great strength, stamina and flexibility. In particular, the vinyasa (see pages 70–73) and sun salutations (see pages 46–53) build a lot of upper body strength. You also begin to notice that your posture improves, not just when you are doing yoga but in the rest of your life too.

The longer-term benefits of Astanga yoga include ease in breathing and efficient, untroubled digestion. All the major body systems respond well to the release of deep-seated tensions; skin, hair and nails reveal the good condition of the inner body by their strong and healthy appearance. Improved sleep quality is also a common and very welcome side effect of any yoga practice. Many people claim to have made miraculous recoveries from illness or injury through Astanga yoga. A powerful physical and mental discipline combined with an uplifting spiritual message can and does bring about extraordinary transformations on many levels.

The psychological benefits

Astanga yoga is challenging; when you first see a demonstration of the practice you may find that you doubt your ability to do all those complicated postures. But with dedicated practice, each posture gradually becomes possible. This can be a fantastic boost to your self-esteem, and can give you a new-found physical confidence and sense of ease within your own body.

People also notice changes in their moods, behaviour and outlook on life after a few months or years of yoga practice. These may start with increased mental energy and an improved ability to concentrate. In time, you may find that Astanga yoga gives you a feeling of inner strength, focus and stability which means that you are better able to cope with stress, and the ups and downs of everyday life.

Over time you also develop better powers of observation, both of the world around you and of yourself. The capacity for clear self-observation is especially significant because it can lead to profound change from within. As you become more sensitive to your inner self, the eight limbs of Patanjali's yoga (see pages 18–19) may begin to speak to you in a different way.

One of the advantages of Astanga yoga is its structure. Because you repeat the same postures in the same order each time, your practice is always consistent. This allows you to use the practice as a way of monitoring how you are feeling on a daily basis; Astanga yoga forms a backdrop that throws into sharp relief even the most subtle emotional and physical changes.

For some people this system of yoga will always remain a primarily physical practice – but for others it becomes a devotional one. Yoga is a spiritual tradition with an extraordinarily rich heritage. You do not need to be a Hindu to embrace this spiritual aspect; you can simply devote your practice to something "higher" than yourself. Patanjali is not specific about who or what this higher force might be. As a result, yoga can have spiritual meaning for any person of any – or no – religious belief.

The potential drawbacks

Although Astanga yoga can bring tremendous benefits, it also poses some difficulties and risks. Learning to do some of the more complicated postures can bring a great sense of accomplishment; but the flip side of the coin is that, if you

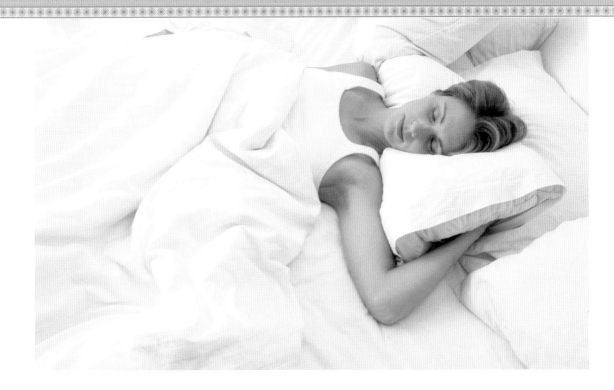

feel that you're not "progressing" quickly enough, you may suffer feelings of obsessiveness and self-criticism, or give up yoga as a hopeless task.

Some Astanga practitioners go through a period of intense practice during which they tend to be obsessive, over-stimulated or even aggressive, and then they mellow into the practice and become calmer. Whether this is a necessary part of the process for some people or an avoidable side effect, I am not sure. However, it is important to know that there is nothing in yogic practice that condones obsessive or excessive practice. If you find that you are putting yourself through pain in order to get into a posture, or you are berating yourself for not being "good enough" at yoga, perhaps it is time to stop and re-think your approach.

If your Astanga yoga practice leads to side effects such as irrational outbursts of anger, fear or aggression (these can be common when you start any intense form of yoga), modify

The benefits of Astanga yoga practice are felt throughout the body. Many people notice that the quality of their sleep improves when they take up yoga.

and soften your practice. Use the modifications to the postures that I suggest (see Chapter 4) and limit your use of the *bandhas* (see page 35) which can over-stimulate your energetic system.

The eminent yoga scholar Georg Feuerstein has said that "Narcissism is as great a danger among Hatha-yogins as it is among bodybuilders." If we don't practice Astanga yoga with care we may end up with inflated, rather than transcended, egos. The purpose of all forms of practice is to increase awareness to the point of a direct experience or an understanding of ultimate reality. We should be wary of deluding ourselves on this journey as there may be many pitfalls along the way.

astanga yoga in daily life

There are strict traditional instructions about how, when, where and for how long you should practise Astanga yoga each day. However, following the spirit rather than the letter of the law may help you to adapt Astanga yoga to fit into your everyday life in a way that enables you to sustain a long-term practice.

Tailoring your practice

One of the distinguishing features of Astanga yoga is that it is hard work. It requires concentration, stamina and tenacity. Although some people have successfully used Astanga yoga to help them through difficult periods, many more have started it with enthusiasm, only to give up when life events make it hard to commit to such an intense practice.

There are two approaches to this issue: you can either approach Astanga yoga as an irreducible set standard to which you apply yourself (with the possibility of regular failure), or you can be flexible in your practice. The latter is my preferred approach because it enables you to tailor yoga to your individual needs and makes it possible for you to keep up a consistent daily practice, even if the content varies.

So, if you can't always practise first thing in the morning or for two hours every day, don't give up yoga! I have devised sequences for those beginning Astanga yoga and those who have a limited amount of time – both are adapted versions of the Primary Series (see pages 118–121).

Traditionally a student must perfect each posture of the series before moving onto the next one. This provides an excellent safety device, slowing students down and ensuring each pose is thoroughly understood before the next is attempted. However, some students will simply be unable to progress beyond a certain pose if they have physical limitations, leaving them for months or years with an incomplete practice. It seems to make sense to modify poses as you go along, making the whole series more accessible to everyone.

The time of day

The traditional time to practise Astanga yoga in India is very early in the morning (before 5am). Early rising is considered to be a sign of discipline, spiritual fervour and devotion. There are practical advantages of starting early: the mind is alert, there are few distractions and in India it is possible to avoid the intense heat of the sun.

Even if it's not realistic for you to practise before 5am, it's a good idea to do yoga first thing in the morning before you start your daily routine. Practising Astanga yoga in the evening is not recommended because you are likely to be less alert and more tired, and your digestive system is processing the food you have eaten during the day. In addition, Astanga yoga can be very stimulating; if you practise in the evening, you may notice that you feel wide awake for hours past your normal bedtime.

Your practice space

You don't need a dedicated yoga space; you just need a room or part of a room in which there is enough space to stretch out when you are lying down, move your arms when you are standing up and accommodate a yoga mat. It helps to do yoga in a warm, peaceful and pleasant environment where there is plenty of light and fresh air (unless this makes the room too cold). Choose a place that is as free from distractions as possible. You can also practise outside, as long as you are not in direct sunlight or the temperature is not too low for comfort. (According to Shri K Pattabhi Jois, you should avoid warming up by jogging or standing in front of a fire if you are cold!)

Don't worry if you don't have an ideal place in which to practise yoga; within about two minutes of starting your practice your attention turns inward and you will be much less conscious of your environment.

Choose a yoga mat that feels comfortable. There are several different types on the market including "sticky", cotton and foam mats. "Sticky" mats are good for helping your feet

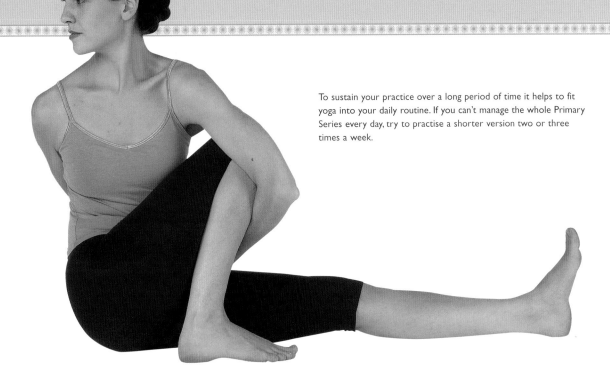

To sustain your practice over a long period of time it helps to fit yoga into your daily routine. If you can't manage the whole Primary Series every day, try to practise a shorter version two or three times a week.

to get a stable grip, cotton mats are comfortable and good at absorbing moisture, and thicker foam mats offer plenty of padding, although some people find them more difficult to balance on.

Duration and frequency

Ideally, one session of Astanga yoga should be practised each day with two rest days a month – practitioners at Mysore (see page 15) traditionally take a break on days of a new or full moon. However, most people who also have a full-time job, and family and social commitments find this schedule too demanding. Try to devise an alternative schedule that you find sustainable. For example, you might be able to do a short practice (see pages 120–121) two or three times a week and the whole Primary Series once a week. Avoid setting yourself unrealistic targets that you can't meet, and avoid practising in an erratic way, for example, doing nothing for a week and then practising the full Primary Series. The latter approach can lead to injury.

Your focus of attention

Because you repeat the same sequence of postures every time you practise Astanga yoga, you have the opportunity to vary the focus of your attention on each occasion. Maintaining a single point of focus throughout a practice provides you with lots of material on which to work, and helps you to explore the subtleties of Astanga yoga. Your point of focus may be a physical one – such as maintaining freedom in your jaw and neck, or being aware of the specific movements of your feet – or it may be a mental focus such as counting the length of each breath.

After your practice

Allow yourself a brief period of time after a practice to let yourself settle and assimilate the benefits of the postures. Don't rush straight from a practice into work or a social engagement – allow yourself time to re-surface. Try to avoid eating immediately after a practice; you may feel very hungry, but wait around 30 minutes if possible.

astanga yoga and you

According to Ayurveda some people are constitutionally well suited to Astanga yoga, whereas others may benefit from a more gentle or nurturing style of yoga. Children, older people, and pregnant and breastfeeding women fall into the latter group. Astanga yoga can be adapted to take account of your constitution and circumstances so that you can still derive the benefits of this system of training.

What is Ayurveda?

Ayurveda is the traditional Indian system of medicine, and it uses yoga as both a preventive and curative tool. According to Ayurveda everyone has a unique constitution that is determined at birth. Your constitution, which influences your physique, health, personality and behaviour, consists of a combination of three *doshas*: *Vata*, *Pitta* and *Kapha*.

Vata is the element of air, *Pitta* is the element of fire and *Kapha* is the element of water. One of these elements usually dominates your constitution, and the other two elements play a less important role. A few people are *tridoshic*, meaning that all three *doshas* are evenly balanced, and a few people seem to have only two elements and none of the third.

If you are considering taking up Astanga yoga, it is worth identifying your dominant *dosha* (see box) and assessing whether this style of yoga is most suited to you. Some people may be constitutionally less suited to Astanga yoga, and either need to learn in a particularly stable and nurturing environment or choose a different style of yoga to practise. Alternatively, if you already practise Astanga yoga, identifying your dominant *dosha* can help you to recognize and tackle any possible problems in your yoga practice, such as burn-out, competitiveness or erratic practise.

The *Vata* constitution

Vata is the element of movement, and people with a *Vata* constitution are attracted to the constant movement of Astanga yoga (a vast majority of the people in Astanga yoga classes are *Vata* types). They quickly become proficient at it because they learn quickly and have light, agile bodies. However, they lack stamina and their practice is often erratic, see-sawing between bursts of enthusiasm and days, weeks or months of recovery. For this reason, Astanga yoga may not always be ideal for *Vata* individuals. If you have a *Vata* constitution, you will benefit more from a gentle, nourishing practice. Adapt your Astanga practice to be slow and steady, and balance it by ensuring that other aspects of your life are grounded and stable, for example, eat regular meals, get plenty of rest, and avoid overwork and an excessively busy lifestyle.

The *Pitta* constitution

Pitta-types are naturally competitive – both with themselves and others – and Astanga yoga is appealing in that it appears to provide a ladder of progress to climb. *Pitta* individuals can derive most benefit from Astanga yoga if they attempt to check their competitive instincts and, instead of treating yoga as a set of goals, approach it as an on-going journey of self-development. Taking care to practise steadily and meticulously is important if you have a *Pitta* constitution because you are prone to over-heating and burning out.

The *Kapha* constitution

Kapha individuals are strong, steady people with good stamina and determination, and because of this they are likely to derive great benefits from an Astanga yoga practice. The dynamic postures make them feel lighter and brighter, and give them a welcome boost of heating energy that inspires and revitalizes them. Astanga yoga counteracts the tendency of the *Kapha* individual to be sluggish.

Children and Astanga yoga

Astanga yoga is not suitable for young children because their bones, joints and organs are not fully formed. The deep stretches and athletic nature of the Primary Series place stress

CHARACTERISTICS OF DIFFERENT *DOSHA* TYPES

	PERSONALITY	BUILD	FACE	SKIN	HAIR
VATA	Learns – and forgets – quickly. Adaptable, but low stamina. Loses interest and often leaves tasks unfinished.	Light, small frame	Oval-shaped	Dry, dusky	Dry, thin, frizzy
PITTA	Highly concentrated, focused and goal achieving. Tendency to burn-out.	Medium	Heart-shaped	Oily, pale, freckles	Thin, fine, oily; often fair/red
KAPHA	Great stamina. Slow on the uptake, but reliable and focused once a task is in hand. Can get stuck in a rut.	Solid and strong	Round or square	Pale, cool	Thick, wavy, lustrous

upon their bodies and increase the risk of stretched ligaments, unstable joints, disturbed hormonal development and future osteoporosis (the same problems that are associated with the early training of gymnasts and dancers). The strict discipline that is required in Astanga yoga is also unsuitable for children. If you would like to do yoga with your child, look for a yoga teacher who is experienced in teaching children or consult a book on the subject (see page 139). Children love exploring their bodies through the practice of yoga, but tend to respond best to yoga when it is presented in an easy and playful style.

Older people and Astanga yoga

Although there are a number of notable exceptions, most Astanga practitioners are in their 20s, 30s or 40s. Astanga yoga is essentially a young person's practice, and older people tend to find it draining rather than invigorating. If you have been practising Astanga yoga for a long time, then you may find you can continue well into later life. However, if you are in your 60s and are thinking about taking up yoga for the first time, you would probably benefit from practising a more gentle style of yoga. This is particularly true if you suffer from a musculoskeletal condition, such as osteoarthritis or osteoporosis. Shri K Pattabhi Jois (see pages 14–15) recommends that older people concentrate on yogic breathing exercises (*pranayama*) rather than posture practice, and that if they do practise Astanga yoga, to omit the vinyasa.

Yoga during menstruation

Traditionally, women are instructed not to practise Astanga yoga while they are menstruating. Although it is easy to dismiss this as outdated, it does make sense on both a physical and an energetic level to rest at this time. Inverted postures, such as headstand and shoulderstand, and semi-inverted postures, such as down-facing dog, are to be avoided because they cause blood to flow back toward the uterus instead of out of the body. On a general level, the heating nature of Astanga yoga (see page 34) is said to be incompatible with menstruation.

Many yoga teachers believe that adapting a yoga practice to the menstrual cycle results in a reduction in menstrual problems, such as premenstrual syndrome and painful periods. They recommend treating menstruation as a time to withdraw and contemplate. Take a few rest days and try practising some gentle, open and passive postures, such as *Baddha Konasana* A (see page 92), during menstruation. Many women feel naturally inclined toward a softer and more introverted

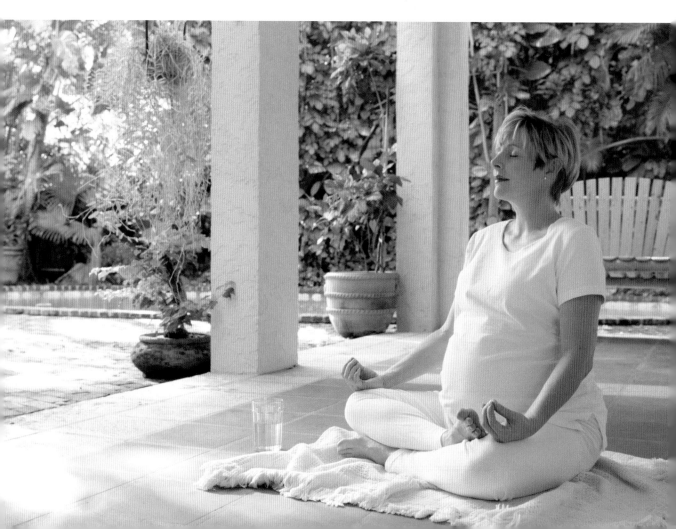

yoga practice during menstruation anyway. You may find yourself able to meditate easily at this time.

If you have irregular, missed or painful periods, or you are experiencing difficulty conceiving, you may be over-exercising and could possibly benefit from a more gentle yoga practice. Do your Astanga yoga practice slowly and gently, omit the vinyasa and perhaps consider a more gentle form of yoga as an alternative.

Yoga during pregnancy

Although I have come across many women who have continued their Astanga yoga practice during pregnancy using lots of modifications, I believe that, in general, Astanga yoga isn't suitable for pregnant women. You should avoid intense exercise, anyway, during the first 14 weeks when pregnancy is not yet established and miscarriage is a possibility. Later on in pregnancy, the Primary Series becomes practically impossible because it consists almost entirely of forward bends.

Throughout pregnancy, your tendons and ligaments are soft and stretchy in preparation for giving birth. Although this makes you supple, over-stretching can cause your joints to become permanently unstable. In addition, increased production of muscle-building hormones as a result of strong exercise can interfere with foetal development.

If you have never done Astanga yoga before, pregnancy is not the time to start. Instead, you will benefit greatly from going to a yoga class specifically for pregnant women in which you will be taught postures and breathing exercises that prepare you mentally and physically for labour and childbirth. Opinions differ as to exactly the best yoga practice for pregnancy, although the consensus is that gentle and relaxing yoga works best. Interestingly, in *Yoga Mala*, Shri K Pattabhi Jois (see pages 14–15) gives instructions to stop all

Tendons and ligaments become soft and stretchy during pregnancy which makes women vulnerable to joint instability caused by overstretching. This is just one of the reasons why the intense practice of Astanga yoga should be avoided if you are pregnant. Practise simple sitting postures and breath exercises instead.

yoga practice from four months of pregnancy except *pranayama* (breathing exercises), *Mahamudra* (a seated "seal" that looks very much like *Janu Sirsasana*; see page 79) and *Padmasana* (lotus position; see page 115). See page 139 for recommended books on yoga during pregnancy.

Post-natal yoga

In the West there is enormous cultural pressure on women to get back to "normal" after having a baby. You may be encouraged to do vigorous exercise in order to re-gain your pre-pregnancy figure as quickly as possible. In my opinion, this seems to be a peculiarly negative approach to motherhood, and one that should be avoided. Not only will you never be the same as you were before (you have just undergone the most profound change possible for a human being!) your baby needs you to be relaxed and nurturing rather than exhausted and muscle-bound.

Post-natal exercise needs to be measured and gentle. If you are breastfeeding, your tendons and ligaments are still soft, and deep stretching is inadvisable. When you stop breastfeeding you may wish to return to the Primary Series (the forward bends and *bandhas* will help you to restore a core of strength in your body), or you may feel, as most mothers do, that combining the demands of Astanga yoga with the duties of parenthood is not really practical in the early years. If you have two spare hours, you may prefer to sleep or relax with your partner! You can start or resume Astanga yoga in the future when your child is older – when the time is right it can be wonderful to return to a demanding practice that allows you to turn deeply inward again.

However, some gentle yoga is beneficial and it can be slotted into your day in short bursts. Realistically, you are unlikely to have more than 15 minutes to yourself at a time in the post-natal period. Use that time to do gentle stretches; focus on keeping your chest open, and your hips and knees narrow. Relaxing on your back with your knees bent and your feet on the floor helps to alleviate low backache. See page 139 for recommended books on post-natal yoga.

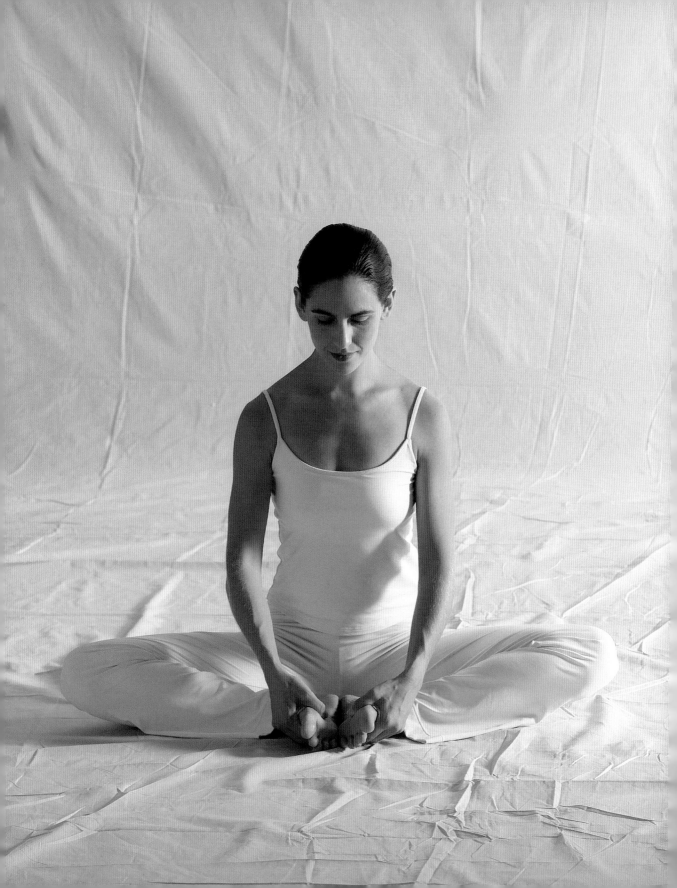

chapter three

basic principles

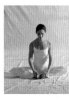

Astanga yoga is not about contortionist gymnastics! Without
an understanding of the fundamental principles of the system
we can do ourselves damage or forego the immense benefits
that we might otherwise experience. This chapter outlines the
basic principles that underpin Astanga yoga and explains the
effects that yoga has on the mind and body. The characteristic
deep breathing and body "locks" are explained in detail, both
from an anatomical and an esoteric point of view. Applying
these basic principles helps to transform the postures in
Chapter 4 from an athletic form of exercise into a real yoga
practice with all its associated benefits for mind, body and
soul. The chapter ends with two *mantra* that are traditionally
chanted at the start and close of a yoga practice.

understanding astanga yoga

Astanga Vinyasa yoga is built on a foundation of core principles that are common to many styles of Hatha yoga, but are given special emphasis in this system. If you have an understanding of these principles, it not only helps you to understand the traditional form of the practice, but also makes it possible to modify the form, if necessary, without losing its essence.

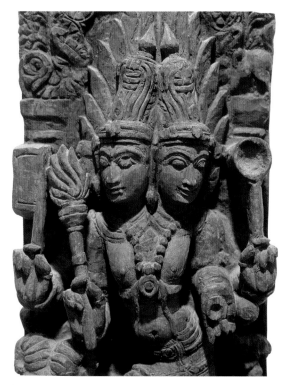

Agni, the Vedic god of fire, is depicted in this southern Indian wood carving dating from the 17th century BCE.

The postures of Astanga yoga are so impressive that we sometimes tend to get carried away with the details of the technique to the exclusion of all else. The core principles that underpin this practice are the combined use of a steady, regular *ujjayi* breath, muscular locks called *bandhas*, the connecting of breath and movement in vinyasa and the steady point of focus known as *drishti*. The combination of these powerful techniques is called *tristana* and it provides the framework for your practice. Although these are all elements practised in other forms of yoga, their combination and emphasis in this practice make it unique. It is these elements that differentiate an Astanga yoga practice from what would otherwise be a kind of stretching or gymnastic routine.

Heat – purification through fire

The cleansing and purifying nature of heat during yoga practice – referred to as *tapas* – is a concept that appears in various different styles of yoga and in many yoga texts. In some styles of yoga, the practice room is heated to a high temperature. In Astanga yoga it is thought that heat must be generated from within.

The heat generated when you practise Astanga yoga is said to have a strong cleansing and purifying effect on your body, and to burn away mental, emotional, physical and spiritual debris. Heat comes from three sources: the athleticism of the movements themselves, the fast-moving pace of an Astanga yoga series and the combined use of *ujjayi* breath and the *bandhas* (see pages 35–39).

On a physical level, heat quickly makes your body much more flexible. When your muscles and joints are very warm they become pliable and soft, and stretch much further than they would do normally. This is important in Astanga yoga because it prevents you from injuring yourself in postures that demand great flexibility. Sweating during yoga practice is purifying because it carries toxins out of your body.

Heat purifies the mind and spirit as well as the physical body. The theory of yoga teaches that human beings exist in a subtle as well as a physical form. The subtle body has its own distinct anatomy consisting of channels (known as *nadis*) and energy centres (known as *chakras*). In the area of the navel is the digestive fire, known as *Agni*. Heat produced during yoga stokes *Agni*, with the result that "impurities", such as emotional blockages and mental patterns, are burnt away, allowing energy to flow freely around the body's subtle anatomy.

Bandhas: the locks of yoga

Bandha is the term that is used in yoga to refer to a muscular contraction or "lock". *Bandhas* produce particular effects on both the physical and the subtle bodies: they increase physical strength, develop muscular control, support your spine and have a quickening effect on the subtle energy. The powerful effect of the upward rise of subtle energy should not be underestimated; in many ways it is what makes this practice physically possible.

In Astanga yoga three *bandhas* are used during posture practice: *mula*, *uddiyana* and *jalandhara bandhas*. Mula and *uddiyana bandha* are held, to some degree, throughout the entire session. In many other schools of yoga, *bandhas* are practised only in association with breathing exercises, *mudra* (seals) and meditation – or by themselves.

Bandhas can be contracted mildly or strongly, or anywhere in between. At first you may only be able to tell the difference between a *bandha* that is either fully engaged or not engaged. If your pelvic floor and low abdominal muscles are weak, for example, you may also find that you can only hold a contraction for a few seconds before your muscles just seem to "slip away". It takes time and practise to use the *bandhas* with great precision.

There are many places in the Primary Series where a movement which is physically challenging or even seemingly impossible becomes easily manageable when you engage the *bandhas*. For example, it's common to feel that your arms are too short or weak to lift your body in many of the lifting poses or to jump through in the vinyasa (see pages 70–73). In these cases, fully engaging the *bandhas* can instantly make you feel lighter and stronger so that a movement becomes possible.

Another benefit of using the lower *bandhas* is that they indirectly increase your breathing capacity. During a normal inhalation, your diaphragm moves down from its arched resting position at the bottom of your ribcage and pushes out your abdomen. When your lower *bandhas* are engaged, your diaphragm can't descend in the usual way so your abdomen doesn't swell outward. Instead, your breath meets resistance and spreads upward and outward through your chest. This causes your lungs to inflate fully and expand the chest muscles (the intercostals) from the inside. This way of breathing is now commonly called "empowered thoracic breathing" and it produces a positive and focused mental state. For more information about breathing and *bandhas*, refer to David Coulter's excellent book, *Anatomy of Hatha Yoga* (see page 139).

Mula bandha: root lock

The Sanskrit word *mula* means "root" and this *bandha* is universally acknowledged as being of great importance in yoga. However, authorities do not seem to agree fully as to the exact technique to be used. There may be some difficulties in translating the terms used. Some texts refer to *mula bandha* as an "anal lock", which is confusing because there is another lock called *ashwini mudra* (the horse seal) which involves the contraction of the anal sphincter but is different from *mula bandha*. In the Astanga yoga Primary Series we are told that *mula bandha* should be contracted throughout the entire practice (if you try to contract the anal sphincter and execute a forward bend, it is virtually impossible to hold). Other authorities describe *mula bandha* as a contraction of the perineal area and, as this is my understanding of the *bandha*, I have described it in more detail below.

Mula bandha consists of the lifting of the pelvic floor muscles. The result is a feeling of core strength in the body, and of mental and physical lightness. "Perineum" is the term used to describe the whole diamond-shaped area of the pelvic floor (see the illustrations on page 37). It is formed of two triangles that are joined by a line between the sitting bones (ischial tuberosities). It is also the term used for the small fibro-muscular nodule at the middle of the pelvic floor into which several muscles insert. It is this area – specifically the central tendon of the perineum – that you need to lift in *mula bandha*.

Practise *mula bandha* with some simple static postures before trying to hold it while moving. At first, the best way to do this is to try to lift everything – the whole diamond-shaped area (see illustrations opposite). The best position in which to do this may be lying on your back on the floor and lifting your hips so that you are in a gentle bridge pose. Squeeze your buttock muscles and pelvic floor while tilting your pubic bone toward the ceiling. Now see if you can keep the same position and gradually release the muscles of your buttocks and thighs a little. If you can keep the lift in the pelvic floor, you are now using a form of *mula bandha* (rather a gross form, but one that can be refined with practice).

You may find that the muscles in this area are quite weak and that it's difficult to hold a contraction at first, but with practice the muscles will become much stronger. Now try to differentiate between the the urogenital triangle at the front of the pelvic floor and the anal triangle at the back. You can do this while sitting upright on a firm flat seat. If you roll forward a little on the seat and try to lift your pelvic floor, you will probably feel the urogenital triangle lift most strongly. If you tilt the pelvis the other way and slump backward slightly, you will find that the anal triangle seems more strongly lifted. Now sit upright and try to gently lift the central tendon of the perineum while leaving the anal triangle soft and relaxed. This is a more subtle version of *mula bandha* and one that can be held throughout *asana* practice with varying degrees of strength. *Mula bandha* probably feels different for men and women, in that women feel the contraction of the front pelvic floor muscles higher up in the body (in the region of the cervix).

Now try practising *mula bandha* while doing a standing forward bend and in down-facing dog (see pages 46–47). To perfect the simultaneous contraction of the front of the pelvic floor and the relaxation of the anus takes time, concentration and practise.

Uddiyana bandha: upward flying lock

In Astanga yoga the term *uddiyana bandha* refers to the lifting of your low abdominal muscles (beneath your naval) to further enhance the action of *mula bandha*, strengthen support for your lower back and force energy upward in the body. In other schools of yoga *uddiyana bandha* describes the total contraction of your abdomen while holding your breath (which obviously limits your ability to do a range of postures).

To contract *uddiyana bandha*, gently draw the muscles beneath your naval in and up. You may find that *mula bandha* spontaneously rises at the same time. Take a few breaths here. Your lower abdomen should stay still when you inhale and exhale, and your chest should inflate on each inhalation. Although *mula bandha* and *uddiyana bandha* are distinct and separate practices, if you concentrate on one, you are often able to do the other one automatically.

Take care that the effort to hold *uddiyana bandha* doesn't produce tension around your diaphragm and the lower part of your ribcage – both of these areas should remain soft throughout.

Jalandhara bandha: throat lock

This is a simple movement that consists of moving your chest toward your chin and your chin toward your chest. This contracts your throat and helps to block the escape of breath and energy through your mouth and nose. In Astanga yoga, you generally perform *jalandhara bandha* spontaneously as a result of the posture that you are in – for example, in any of the shoulderstanding postures (see pages 105–109), when your throat is naturally constricted as a result of the angle between your head and chest. You use a gentle *ujjayi* breath during *jalandhara bandha*.

POSITION OF *MULA BANDHA* IN WOMEN

POSITION OF *MULA BANDHA* IN MEN

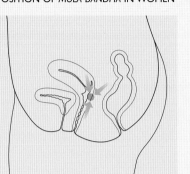
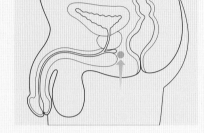

Engaging *mula bandha* during Astanga yoga practice makes many postures more manageable. These two cross-sections of the female and male reproductive systems show the position of *mula bandha*. It is slightly higher in women than in men.

THE FEMALE PERINEUM

THE MALE PERINEUM

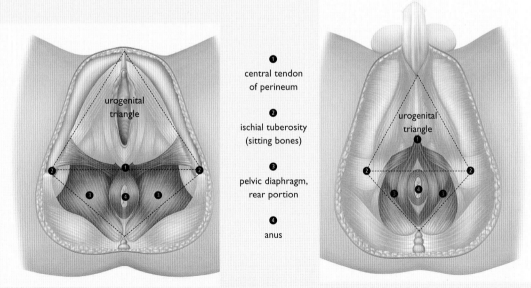

1 central tendon of perineum

2 ischial tuberosity (sitting bones)

3 pelvic diaphragm, rear portion

4 anus

Engaging *mula bandha* involves contracting the perineum, a diamond-shaped area formed of two triangles that are subdivided by a line between the sitting bones. These two cross-sections show the anatomy of the perineum in women and men.

UJJAYI BREATH

Sit upright in a comfortable position and take a few normal preparatory breaths. Now inhale and exhale through your mouth, making a long "hah" sound on each exhalation, as if you were trying to steam up a mirror. Notice how this feels in your throat. Close your mouth, inhale normally through your nose and try to replicate the sound "hah" while exhaling through your nose. You should be making a gentle hissing noise, similar to the one you hear when you put a shell to your ear to listen to the sea. Do this a few times. Now try to make roughly the same sound when you inhale as when you exhale. The sensation is slightly higher up in your throat on the inhalation than on the exhalation and the sound is of a slightly different quality. Do this for a few more breaths and then relax and return to breathing normally again.

As you become more familiar with *ujjayi* breathing, check that each breath you take is of equal length, that your inhalations are the same length as your exhalations (count silently to yourself), that there is no hint of strain or tension in your jaw or tongue, no change in pressure as you breathe and no gasping or sighing sounds.

At first you may feel that you have to concentrate hard to maintain *ujjayi* breath and that it requires effort to breathe in this way. However, with regular practice, *ujjayi* breath becomes automatic and you will find you can easily maintain it throughout your yoga practice.

Ujjayi: the victorious breath

Astanga yoga continuously uses only one *pranayama* (breathing practice). This is *ujjayi* breath, meaning victorious breath. *Ujjayi* breath is practised throughout the entire sequence of Astanga yoga postures without a break. It consists of the narrowing of the air passages in your throat which enables precise control of the flow of air into and out of your body.

Astanga yoga postures are very challenging and *ujjayi* breathing can greatly enhance your ability to do them. It increases your lung capacity (which helps you to breathe fully, deeply and steadily even when you are not practising yoga), it creates a feeling of heat in your body which enables your muscles to stretch without injury (if you do the same poses without *ujjayi* breath, your body doesn't seem to become as hot or as supple), and it increases the detoxifying nature of the poses. *Ujjayi* breath also has mental benefits: the soft sounds are soothing and create a steady rhythm to accompany your practice, and they also give you the focus that you need to turn your concentration inward and reach a meditative state.

If you breathe normally during exercise, your breathing rate naturally speeds up as your body copes with the exertion. If you practise *ujjayi* breath, however, you can control the length and pressure of your exhalation very precisely, and this enables you to maintain breath control and avoid panting, even during intense exercise. An experienced Astanga yoga practitioner is able to execute the entire Primary Series while breathing evenly and rhythmically throughout. This facilitates a stillness of mind even during the most challenging of physical postures.

Astanga yoga without *ujjayi* breath makes the postures more akin to a gymnastic workout. Quite simply, the continuous, steady flow of *ujjayi* breath is what makes your Astanga practice into yoga.

If you practise *ujjayi* breath while applying the lower *bandhas* (see pages 35–37), you'll find that this quickly generates heat within your body. Internal heat (see page 34) is a characteristic trait of Astanga yoga practice. In yogic teaching there are two types of *prana* (energy) which flow in opposite directions in the body: *prana* which flows upward and *apana* which flows downward. When you apply all the *bandhas* and use *ujjayi* breathing, the downward force of *apana* is pushed upward and the upward force of *prana* is pushed downward. This creates a combustible force of energy in the centre of the body at a point known as *Agni* (fire) where heat is created. Experiment by breathing naturally and then doing a few rounds of *ujjayi* breathing with the lower *bandhas* applied and see if you feel any warmer – the effect can be almost instantaneous!

Drishti

The term *drishti* comes from the word *dris* in Sanskrit meaning "to see". It is usually translated as "gazing point" and refers to the direction in which you look during each posture, but *drishti* can also mean intelligence or the direction of one's thoughts. The nine traditional *drishti* points are: *Nasagrai* – the tip of the nose; *Broomadhya* – the third eye (*ajna chakra*); *Nabi chakra* – the navel; *Hastagrai* – the hand; *Padhayoragrai* – the toes; *Parsva* – left; *Parsva* – right; *Angusta ma dyai* – the thumb; and *Urdhva or antara* – upward.

Gazing at a particular point, such as the tip of your nose, helps you to focus and concentrate deeply during a posture. It also acts as a natural balancing aid. Each posture in Astanga yoga has a specific *drishti* point on which you focus both your eyes and mind – these are indicated for each posture in Chapter 4. If you find that a particular *drishti* causes discomfort or tension in your neck, try concentrating mentally on the *drishti* while looking at your nose or gazing straight ahead. I have done this in the photographs on pages 78–82 – instead of looking at my toes I am gazing at the tip of my nose. You may need to make a few temporary alterations to the practical performance of the *drishti* until you are able to manage them without undue strain.

Empowered thoracic breathing (see page 35), the term used by David Coulter in *The Anatomy of Hatha Yoga*, describes the deep chest breathing used during vigorous *asana* practice. It is enhanced by the use of *ujjayi* and *bandha* techniques.

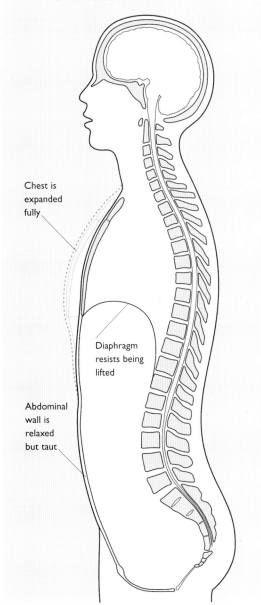

EMPOWERED THORACIC BREATHING

Chest is expanded fully

Diaphragm resists being lifted

Abdominal wall is relaxed but taut

meditation in movement

One of the most therapeutic and beautiful aspects of Astanga yoga is the way in which it can become a moving form of meditation. The concept of meditation in movement is common in spiritual traditions, for example, walking meditation or t'ai chi. Once you have learned the postures of the Primary Series you can repeat them without "thinking" and this has a deeply soothing effect on your mind. It enables you to focus inward and draw your attention to the steady rhythmic sound of your breathing.

The fifth, sixth and seventh limbs of yoga (see pages 18–19) are sense withdrawal, concentration and meditation. Astanga yoga encompasses all these elements within the practice. Sense withdrawal is understood as a process of turning the normally outward focus of the senses inward so that you listen to the sound of your breath, use your eyes to focus on the gazing points (*drishti*; see page 39) and feel the movement of your body. Sense withdrawal induces a state of concentration in which all your faculties are turned to the object of focus – the series you are moving through. Meditation occurs spontaneously from concentration as your focus deepens. You are able to become totally absorbed by it, to the point where you no longer differentiate yourself from the object of your focus which is *samadhi*, the eighth limb: the superconscious state. There are varying degrees of the meditative state – you may frequently slip into a mild form of this kind of meditation when walking. In fact, a well known cure for unsolved problems is a "turn around the block". Repetitive movements can free the mind and make space for it to expand limitlessly.

Stilling your mind

If you are experienced at practising the Primary Series, you may be familiar with the mind state that it can produce. It feels a bit like going into automatic pilot – not in a mindless and dull way, but in a deeply introspective and thoughtful way. Part of your mind becomes detached from the process of doing the postures, and you become able to observe yourself with an objective and unblinking "gaze". One result of this is that the usual background "chatter" of thoughts in your mind disappears and is replaced by a sense of peace, stillness and tranquillity. You may also find that when you lie down to rest at the end of your practice you experience the blissful state of a mind unencumbered with thoughts. Your mind is at ease and resting with your body, yet also fully awake and conscious.

There are ways that you can experience the meditative aspects of Astanga yoga as fully as

You may find that you enter a meditative state naturally when you lie down in corpse pose at the end of your yoga practice.

VINYASA - THE CONNECTING THREAD

One of the defining characteristics of Astanga yoga is that all of the postures are linked by a sequence of movements known in Sanskrit as vinyasa (meaning the order, movement or position of things). These movements provide the connecting thread between the postures, and make the practice of yoga fluid and seamless, which in turn facilitates a calm and meditative state of mind.

Vinyasa also provide important counterposes (without them the postures would make an odd and uncomfortable sequence) in the Primary Series. In particular, the up-facing dog posture in the vinyasa is a strong backbend that forms a counterpose to the huge array of forward bends in the Primary Series. The vinyasa can be thought of as a way of wiping the slate clean – by stretching your body out and realigning your spine – between each posture. Another way of looking at the vinyasa is as the flesh on the bones of the postures. The *Yoga Kurunta* (see page 12) reputedly says: "Oh yogi, don't do yoga without vinyasa".

Vinyasa is inextricably linked with breath. The regular rhythm of the breath dictates the speed and duration of the movements – the two uniting to form a harmonious whole. Meditation on the breath is one of the simplest and most rewarding meditation practices and it is inherent in Astanga yoga; you just need to listen for the sound of each breath, like listening to an internal clock.

possible. First, it helps to release yourself from the pressure to perform – yoga is not about a perfect or spectacular display of athletic expertise. Don't worry about how you look to other people. Concentrate on the internal aspects of yoga – think of it as a way to come back inside yourself. Second, focus on the pace, duration and quality of your breath – it is this that connects your mind with your body and acts as a driving force in the movement of *prana* (see page 38). Your breath is the key to stilling your mind. If you listen carefully, your breath will tell you everything you need to know.

Generally speaking, when you are struggling with a posture your breathing becomes rough and uneven. Prioritizing the quality of your breath over the intensity of your effort is a good way to develop the meditative quality of your practice and the depth and ease of your breathing.

Working slowly

When you first start Astanga yoga you will probably find that it is difficult to reach a meditative state of mind because the postures are so physically challenging. In the early stages, you will find yourself pushing and pulling, huffing and puffing, and incapable of much refinement of your breath or posture. At a later stage, however, you will find that a transformation occurs. You will notice a feeling of lightness and ease in a few postures, which in time spreads to others. Very accomplished practitioners are able to find lightness and ease in every pose most times they practise. They appear to be floating through the whole sequence with delicate care and precision, and report great mental clarity and calm.

If you are a beginner, be patient. Practise at your own pace. Don't let anyone else suck you into a contest to get to the next pose or series, and don't worry too much about where you are going – just be aware of where you are at!

If you are particularly interested in the meditative aspect of Astanga, then it may be useful to do an "easy" practice every now and then; perhaps just the Sun Salutations (see pages 46–53) – ten of each as a way to get into a steady rhythm. At the end of your practice session rest for a few minutes longer than you think you need to – let your mind be at peace in that deeply relaxed state.

opening and closing *mantra*

At the beginning and end of an Astanga yoga practice it is traditional to recite an opening and a closing *mantra* in Sanskrit. These are prayers that express the wish for healing and prosperity, and acknowledge the role of teachers, specifically Patanjali, in the yoga lineage.

The opening *mantra* is composed of two *slokas* (stanzas or verses) from different sources. The first four lines come directly from the first verse of the *Yoga Taravali*, attributed to Adi Sankara, who wrote many commentaries and texts around 700CE. The *Taravali* is an interesting text on yoga and has been recently published in a translation by TKV Desikachar and his son Kausthub from the original dictation given by Krishnamacharya (see pages 14–15). These words are presented as a humble acknowledgement to the long tradition of teachers who have come before us; a traditional Indian custom to set an auspicious tone for the practice to come. The poison of *samsara* is the misery of conditioned existence, all the problems we face; mental, physical and spiritual, which can be removed by yoga.

The second part seems to come from a longer prayer to Patanjali, widely recited and probably dating back to the 18th century. Patanjali, as the author of the *Yoga Sutras*, is seen as the chief among great teachers and in this *sloka* as an incarnation of Adisesa (Siva). He is described in a symbolic incarnation as white, with a thousand heads; gods are often represented with a many-headed cobra rising behind their heads as a protective canopy. He is holding the conch, used as a musical instrument to ward off demons and representing infinite space. The discus is a spinning wheel of light (a *chakra*), symbolic of the cycle of life and death and also of infinite time. The sword represents wisdom, knowledge and discrimination battling against ignorance. BKS Iyengar quotes this same verse as an invocatory prayer both at the beginning of his seminal text *Light on Yoga* and in his more recent *Light on the Yoga Sutras of Patanjali* (see page 139).

The closing *mantra* is derived from the popular Indian epic *The Ramayana*. The translation given here is very literal. Cows and Brahmins are regarded as sacred and hence the prayer for their prosperity. Happiness, health and well-being are wished upon all of mankind and the natural world. People in positions of power are urged to follow the "right path" and do their duty by ruling wisely and well.

The sacred syllable OM is repeated at the beginning and end of both of the *mantra*. This is the usual practice, OM being regarded as the root *mantra* for all others. The repetition of this one syllable alone is said to be capable of bringing about spiritual transcendence. It is a marvellous, resonant sound creating a deep vibration throughout the body that lifts the spirits. According to tradition the sound of OM is the sound of the universe – and we need only to listen to be able to hear it within our hearts.

The *mantra* make a clear start and end to your practice, they enclose and envelop it, creating a special space in which your practice happens. They are an effective way of separating yoga time from the rest of your life; they also make yoga into a ritual, and give it its due weight and respect.

You will need a teacher to help you learn the *mantra*. The traditional way of reciting the *mantra* is in the characteristic flat delivery of the Brahmin priests. However, I have also heard more melodious and even sing-along renditions by some teachers and students of Astanga yoga. Regardless of the style in which the *mantra* are recited, the sound of the Sanskrit language is said to have a holy quality (much like the idea of Latin being sacred in European culture). Even if you don't understand what you are chanting, the simple act of reciting the words creates a positive force.

It is not essential to recite the *mantra*. They are part of the Hindu teachers' tradition, but this may not be meaningful to you. You may prefer to replace the *mantra* with prayers from your own religious or spiritual tradition, or with a positive affirmation that has personal significance.

ॐ

वन्दे गुरूणां चरणारविन्दे
सन्दर्शित स्वास सुखाव बोधे ।
निः श्रेयसं जाङ्गलिकायमाने
संसार हालाहल मोहशांत्यै ॥

आबाहु पुरुषाकारं
शंखचक्रासि धारिणम् ।
सहस्र शिरसं श्वेतं
प्रणमामि पतञ्जलिम् ॥

ॐ

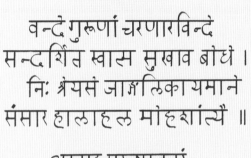

Opening *mantra*

Om
To calm the delirium caused by the
poison of *samsara*, I venerate the lotus
feet of the masters, which awaken
the joy of witnessing the Self.
They are the very best
doctors against poison.

I bow to Patanjali, who is white
and has a thousand heads and who,
with a man's body up to his arms,
holds conch, discus and sword.
Om

ॐ

स्वस्ति प्रजाभ्यः परिपालयन्तां
न्यायेन मार्गेण महीं महीशाः ।
गोब्राह्मणेभ्यः शुभमस्तु नित्यं
लोकासमस्ता सुखिनो भवंतु ॥

ॐ

Closing *mantra*

Om
May all creatures be well!
May the rulers of the earth protect
the world by the right path.
May cows and Brahmins always
be prosperous.
May the whole world
always be happy.
Om

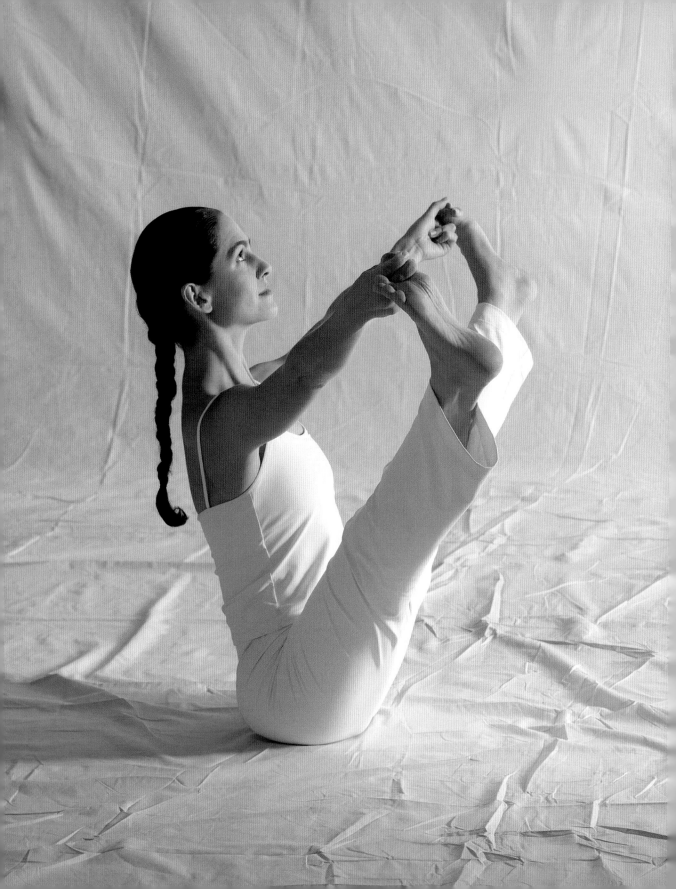

astanga vinyasa postures

This chapter contains photographs and instructions for each of the postures in the Primary Series in the correct order. For every pose I have suggested one or more modifications that you may like to try if the classical pose is too difficult. The series is divided into four parts. The sun salutations are both the warm-up and the core of the practice as they appear in the form of vinyasa throughout the series. Standing postures develop stamina and stability. Seated postures deepen the practice, and fine tune the body and mind. The fourth and finishing sequence is used to restore balance and harmony at the end of the practice. For your ease of reference I have also given the whole series in sequence in thumbnail-sized pictures on pages 122–129. In addition, I have suggested a short practice for beginners and another which can be done by people of all levels to make a balanced 40–50 minute practice when you don't have time to do the whole series. Please make sure that you read chapters 3 and 4 before starting any practice in this book. They give you the background information that you need to do the practice safely and with maximum benefit.

surya namaskara A

SURYA = sun; NAMASKARA = salutation

This is the first full sun salutation of Astanga Vinyasa yoga. Repeat the sequence five times at the beginning of your practice to warm up your body. Do more if you feel cold, or less if you are a beginner.

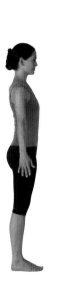
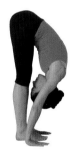
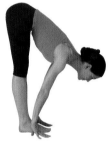

Start with your feet together and your arms lengthening at your sides. This is *Samasthiti*.

1: Inhale, lift your arms overhead, bringing your palms together.

2: Exhale, fold forward at your hips, placing your hands on the floor on either side of the feet. This is *Uttanasana*.

3: Inhale, lift and open your chest. Look forward, leaving your hands on the floor.

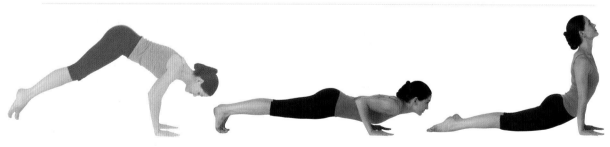

4: Exhale, jump back.

5: Bend your elbows to lower your body so that it is parallel to the floor. Look forward. This is *Chaturanga*.

6: Inhale, roll over on your toes and push into up-facing dog. This is *Urdhva Mukha Svanasana*.

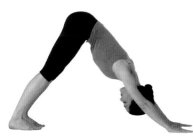

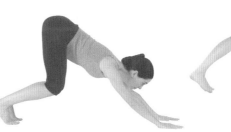

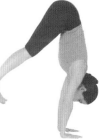

7: Exhale, press your hips up, shoulders broad, and roll over your toes into down-facing dog. Hold for five breaths. This is *Adho Mukha Svanasana*.

8: Inhale, look at the space between your hands and prepare to jump.

9: Lift your hips high as you draw your legs into the space between your hands.

☀ Breathe fluidly and evenly throughout *Surya Namaskara* despite the physical effort involved. Synchronize breath and movement. The breathing pattern is to inhale on upward or opening movements, and exhale on forward-bending movements.

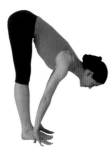

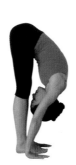

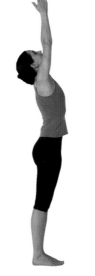

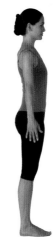

10: Lift your chest and look up.

11: Exhale, draw your head toward your shins. This is *Uttanasana*.

12: Inhale, bring your body back up to standing with your arms overhead.

13: Exhale, return to the starting position: *Samasthiti*.

surya namaskara A – modifications

SURYA = sun; NAMASKARA = salutation

Surya Namaskara A requires quite a bit of strength and flexibility. Rather than forcing your body into a pose, try one of these modifications if you feel stiff or weak.

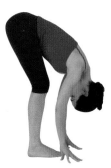 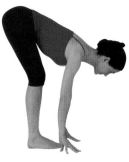 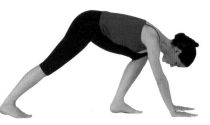

🔴 1: If you can't fold forward with straight legs, bend them. The lengthening of your spine is more important than the stretching of your hamstrings.

2: If your legs were bent in the last pose, keep them bent as you lift your chest in this pose.

3: If you can't jump back into *Chaturanga*, walk back until your body has warmed up or you have built up more strength.

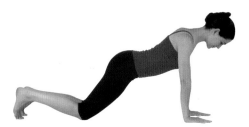 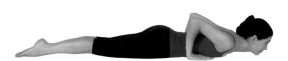

4: If it is difficult to hold *Chaturanga*, drop your knees to the floor first and then lower your chest.

5: Make sure you lower your body as a unit rather than your letting your hips come down first followed by your chest – this puts stress on your lower back.

⊙ Because the sun salutations form the basis of Astanga Vinyasa yoga, it is important that your practice is strong, gentle and safe. According to Patanjali (see pages 18–19) every posture should have the dual qualities of strength and softness: *sthira sukha asanam*. Don't be in a rush to complete the sun salutations and, if there is a posture that you find difficult, use a modification. If you don't build good technique in these preliminary sequences, you risk injuring yourself. Practise with patience.

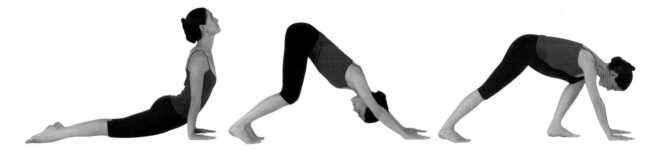

6: If you find up-facing dog tough on your lower back or shoulders, keep your knees on the floor and tilt your pubic bone firmly down toward the floor as you lift up.

7: You can take pressure off your legs in down-facing dog by bending your knees. This helps you to stretch your back more. Do this until you have built up more leg flexibility.

8: You can step forward into the standing pose instead of jumping.

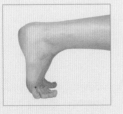
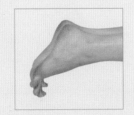
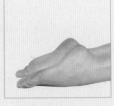

These pictures show rolling over the toes from *Chaturanga* into *Urdhva Mukha Svanasana* (up-facing dog). You need to develop quite a bit of flexibility in your feet and toes to do this well, but it makes a smoother transition than "flipping" the feet over one at a time. Reverse the process to get from *Urdhva Mukha Svanasana* into *Adho Mukha Svanasana* (down-facing dog).

surya namaskara B

SURYA = sun; NAMASKARA = salutation

This is the second sun salutation of Astanga Vinyasa yoga; it should be repeated five times after *Surya Namaskara* A. It introduces an asymmetric movement (the warrior) in steps 7 and 11.

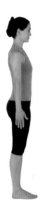 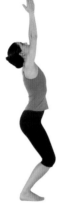 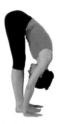 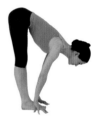

Stand with your feet together and your arms lengthening at your sides. This is *Samasthiti*.

1: Inhale, bend your knees, lift your arms overhead bringing your palms together. Look toward your thumbs. This is *Utkatasana*.

2: Exhale, fold forward at your hips, placing your hands on the floor on either side of the feet. This is *Uttanasana*.

3: Inhale, lift and open your chest. Look forward, leaving your hands on the floor.

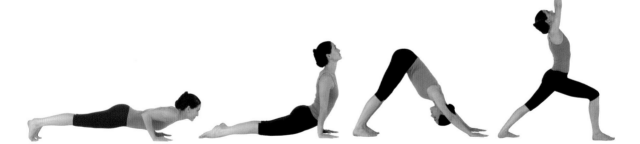

4: Exhale, jump back. Bend your elbows to lower your body so that it is parallel to the floor. Look forward. This is *Chaturanga*.

5: Inhale, roll over on your toes and push your body into up-facing dog. This is *Urdhva Mukha Svanasana*.

6: Exhale, press your hips up and broaden your shoulders to move into down-facing dog. Hold for five breaths. This is *Adho Mukha Svanasana*.

7: Inhale, turn your left heel in and step your right foot forward between your hands. Lift your torso and take your arms overhead, palms together. Look up.

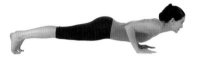

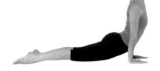

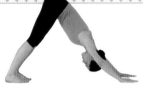

8: Exhale, lower your hands to the floor and step back into *Chaturanga*, lowering your chest and lifting your gaze.

9: Inhale, roll on to the tops of your feet, push your chest forward, draw your shoulders back and down. Straighten your arms in up-facing dog.

10: Exhale, press your hips back and up and roll over your toes into down-facing dog.

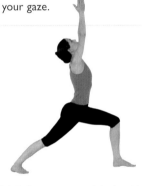

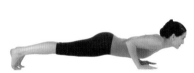

13: Inhale, roll forward onto the tops of your feet straightening your arms and lifting your chest in up-facing dog.

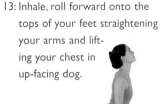

11: Inhale, turn your right heel in and step your left foot forward between your hands. Lift your torso and take your arms overhead, palms together. Look up.

12: Exhale, lower your hands to the floor on either side of your left foot and step back. Lower your chest to the floor and look forward.

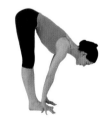

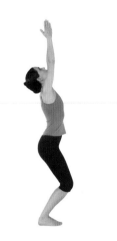

14: Exhale, draw your hips back into down-facing dog, broaden your shoulders and stay for five deep breaths.

15: Inhale, look at the space between your hands and jump forward to land your feet here. Keep your chest open. Gaze at horizon level.

16: Exhale, fold forward at your hips and draw your nose toward your shins.

17: Inhale, bend your knees, lift your body with your arms overhead and your palms together. Look at your thumbs. Exhale, come back to *Samasthiti*.

surya namaskara B – modifications

Most of the modifications for *Surya Namaskara* B are the same as for A. The adaptations here are designed to help you get into *Virabhadrasana* (warrior pose) in steps 7 and 11, and to ease your neck and shoulders.

The sun salutation B sequence really does get you warmed up fully and the addition of the warrior pose adds a new challenge. Your primary focus should be the quality of the vinyasa; you don't want to be staggering from pose to pose gasping for breath. Modify the postures to suit you, and work towards an even and steady breath throughout. When you are ready, you can gradually replace the modifications with the full postures.

Several difficulties with the warrior arise from the stepping forward movement from down-facing dog – this can be difficult at first. You need to use your abdominal strength to help lift your hip high and bring your leg well forward (it's important to use the *bandhas* here). You also need strength when you step back again so that you don't let the whole of your lower back sag. Often, for beginners, your foot will hit the floor well in front of the space between your hands. If this is the case you may need to literally take hold of your foot with one hand and help step it forward. Be aware of the supporting role of your back leg, see if you can keep the instep high off the floor to help support your inner knee.

Even if you can complete the step through, it's common to automatically hold your breath on this movement. There are various possible breathing variations for this move but I recommend the following: in its full form *Surya Namaskara* B requires you to step forward and lift into warrior pose on a single inhalation. Even if you can manage one or two rounds of this, your breath may become very strained by the fourth or fifth round. To maintain an even flow of breath, it is preferable to add an extra breath rather than to struggle or hold your breath. So, after down-facing dog, inhale, turn in your left heel and step forward with your right foot. Exhale. Now take an extra inhalation and lift your arms over your head with your palms together. (Don't forget the *bandhas*, they help to lift you lightly.) You can look up, but if this causes you neck discomfort, modify the pose by looking straight ahead (see opposite). Exhale, lower your hands to the floor and step back into *Chaturanga*. Continue *Surya Namaskara* B as normal.

❸ Sun salutations occur in many forms of yoga and there is a lot of variation in how the postures are performed. For example, in Astanga yoga it's traditional to jump rather than step your feet backward and forward. For an accomplished practitioner, this jump is feather-light, graceful and soft. Beginners may need to build up their strength before they can achieve this.

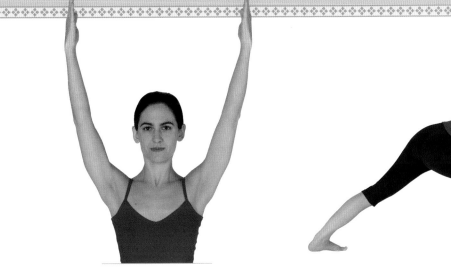

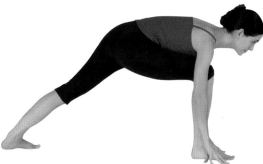

Warrior pose demands strength and flexibility in your chest and shoulders, and bringing your palms together is potentially problematic because it can close the upper part of your chest making your inhalation short as you move into the posture. A solution which helps to maintain the quality of your breath is to open your hands to shoulder-width apart. You may need to do this for some months before you bring your palms together. If you have neck problems, look forward rather than up.

If it is difficult to lift into warrior pose using the breathing modification that I suggest on page 52, simply step forward from down-facing dog and hold that position for one breath. This is a good compromise to start with as it is easier to keep your breath even without lifting up into the full warrior pose. Once you have established this and it is becoming easy, add the full warrior back in again. The key is to build up slowly and carefully – you need good technique to last you through the practice.

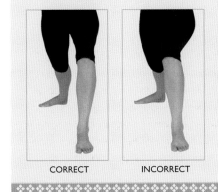

CORRECT   INCORRECT

Take good care of your knees throughout this sequence. Make sure that they track straight over the toes at all times (see left) and that, particularly in *Utkatasana* and the warrior postures (*Virabhadrasana*), they are not under strain. Don't let your knee collapse inward (see right). Keep your foot well grounded and your hips square to the front. This should help to draw your knee directly over your ankle, and you will feel secure and stable in the pose.

padangusthasana

PADA = foot; ANGUSTHA = big toe; ASANA = posture

This deep forward bend produces an intense stretch through the back of your body. Let your pelvis rotate forward and keep your torso soft, especially around your shoulders. Keep your feet stable and relaxed.

Inhale, step or jump your feet hip-width apart. Exhale, put your hands on your hips. Inhale, lift your chest, roll your shoulders back and look up. Exhale, fold forward at your hips, hold your big toes with your index and middle fingers (thumbs on top). Your elbows should be out to the sides, your legs straight, your knees and thigh muscles engaged, and your head and neck relaxed. Lift the *bandhas*. Inhale, look up, open your chest as fully as possible while holding your toes. Exhale, fold forward and stay for five breaths. Inhale, lift and lengthen your spine and look forward. Go straight into the next posture: *Padahastasana*.

✿ Nose

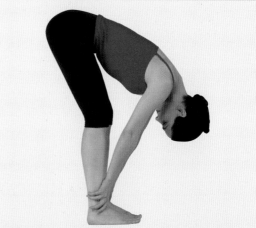

🌸 If it is too difficult or painful to reach your toes with straight legs, you can bend your knees, keeping your back long and your knees tracking forward over your toes. An alternative modification is to rest your hands on your shins or wherever you can comfortably reach (with your legs straight or bent).

padahastasana

PADA = foot; HASTA = hand; ASANA = posture

Bringing the hands and feet together in this way has a curiously reassuring effect. Find a position for your hands that allows you to release the weight of your body through your feet and hands to the floor.

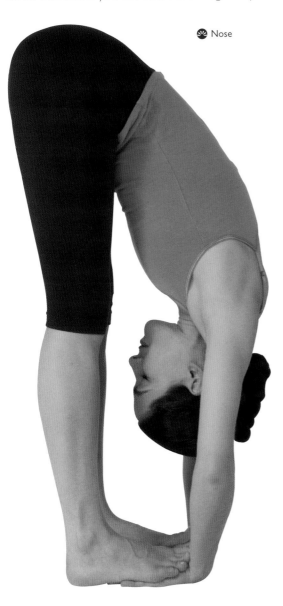

✴ Nose

Exhale, fold forward at your hips and place your hands under your feet, palms to soles, toes to wrists. Inhale, lift your chest and look forward. Exhale, fold fully forward and take five deep breaths. Inhale, lengthen your spine, open your chest and look forward. Exhale, put your hands on your hips. Keep your back flat and your legs straight. Inhale, come back up to standing. Exhale, step or jump your feet together.

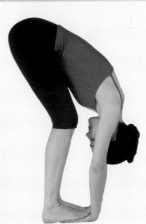

⚜ If you can't put your hands under your feet, bend your knees – this will ease the strain on your lower back. Alternatively, keep your legs straight and just bring your hands as low down your legs as is comfortable.

utthita trikonasana

UTTHITA = extended; TRI = three; KONA = angle; ASANA = posture
This sideways stretch illustrates the importance of the *bandhas* in sustaining a standing
posture without strain. Your back lengthens and your shoulders become free and wide.

Inhale, step or jump your feet one leg-length apart, making a quarter turn to your
right as you do so (to face the long edge of your mat). At the same time, lift your
arms to shoulder height, palms face down. Exhale, turn out your right foot and
slightly turn in the toes of your left foot. Fold deeply into your right hip and take
hold of your right toe with your first two fingers. Keep your legs long and strong,
supporting your spine with the *bandhas*. Reach up with your left arm
and roll open your chest. Turn your head to look at your upper
thumb. Lengthen sideways – lift and roll back your right thigh
and keep your left hip drawn back. Stay for five breaths.
Inhale, come up, secure the *bandhas*. Bring your feet parallel.
Exhale, repeat on your left side by turning out your left
foot, turning your right toes in and folding deeply to
your left. Stay for five breaths. Inhale, come up and go
straight into the next posture: *Parivritta Trikonasana*.

✺ Hand

🌑 If you can't reach your toes without bending your front knee or
folding your body forward a long way, a better option is to place
your hand on your shin instead. Concentrate on keeping your chest
open and in line with your right leg.

parivritta trikonasana

PARIVRITTA = revolved; TRI = three; KONA = angle; ASANA = posture

If the position of your pelvis is right, the rest of this pose will flow easily. Square your hips to the front of your mat and keep them stable as you enter the twist.

Exhale, turn your right foot out by 90 degrees and your left foot in by about 45 degrees. Draw your hips square to the back of your mat, rotating your body to face over your right thigh. Fold forward to place your left hand on the floor on the outer side of the right foot as you lift your right arm to the sky and rotating your torso as fully as possible. Look at your upper thumb. Lengthen your entire torso and broaden your shoulders. Press your back heel firmly to the floor. Press your left hip forward and your right hip back to keep them parallel. Stay for five breaths. Inhale, come up, extending your arms to the sides and turning your feet parallel. Exhale, turn your left foot out by 90 degrees and your right foot in by about 45 degrees. Fold forward to place your right hand on the floor this time. Stay for five breaths. Inhale, come up, extending your arms to the sides and bringing your feet parallel. Exhale, step or jump your feet back together turning to face the front of your mat.

✿ Hand

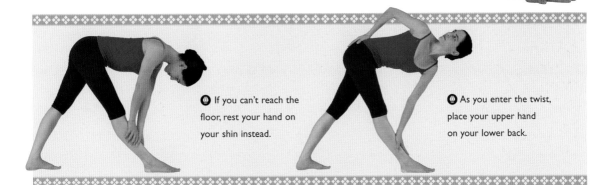

❂ If you can't reach the floor, rest your hand on your shin instead.

❂ As you enter the twist, place your upper hand on your lower back.

utthita parsvakonasana

UTTHITA = extended; PARSVA = side; KONA = angle; ASANA = posture

This deep lunging pose opens your thighs and the sides of your torso. Take care over the position of the bent knee in this pose – if your hips are tight, it will tend to drift forward.

Inhale, step or jump your feet more than a leg-length apart, turning a quarter to your right as you go and lifting your arms to shoulder height. Exhale, turn your right foot out by 90 degrees and your left foot in slightly. Bend your right knee to a deep lunge, knee directly above your ankle. Lower your right hand to the outer side of your right foot, palm to the floor. Stretch your left arm over your head to make a diagonal line from heel to fingertips. Stay for five breaths. Inhale, come up, turn your feet parallel, arms extended to the sides at shoulder height. Exhale, repeat on the other side. Stay for five breaths. Inhale, come up, bring your feet parallel, arms extended to the sides. Go straight into the next posture: *Parivritta Parsvakonasana*.

🌸 Hand

🌼 If you can't get your hand on the floor, place your forearm on your thigh instead. Then, as in the full version of the pose, roll your torso open as you stretch your other arm in the air.

parivritta parsvakonasana

PARIVRITTA = revolved; PARSVA = side; KONA = angle; ASANA = posture

This powerful twist stimulates your internal organs, rotates your spine and challenges your breath. Maintain some weight on your back leg to help you balance.

Exhale, turn your right foot out by 90 degrees and your left foot in by 45 degrees. Bend your right knee to a deep lunge, knee directly above your ankle. Maintain a deep abdominal strength through the *bandhas* and revolve your torso so that you can place your left elbow on the outer side of your right thigh and your left hand on the floor. Keep your back foot well planted on the floor and lift your right arm overhead so that there is a diagonal line from heel to fingertips. Stay for five breaths. Inhale, come up and bring your feet parallel. Exhale, turn out your left foot and repeat on the other side. Stay for five breaths and then inhale, come up slowly and bring your feet parallel. Exhale, step or jump your feet together and come back to the front of your mat in *Samasthiti* (see page 46).

🌸 Hand (or upward if you have your hands in prayer pose)

🌸 If you can't rotate your body enough to get your hand to the floor, bring your left elbow to the outer side of your thigh and bring your palms together in prayer pose.

🌸 It may feel easier to come into the posture by initially dropping your back knee to the floor in order to draw your arm across your thigh. You can straighten your leg as soon as you have established the twist.

prasarita padottanasana A

PRASARITA = spread out; PADA = foot; UTTANA = intense stretch; ASANA = posture

This full stretch for the backs of the legs helps you to feel the essential support of the *bandhas*. They enable you to release your body forward effortlessly, reducing tension in your shoulders and neck.

Inhale, step or jump your feet apart, turning a quarter to your right as you go so that you face the long side of your mat. Bring your feet parallel and your arms to shoulder height. Exhale, put your hands on your hips. Inhale, lift your chest, look upward, drop your tailbone and lift the *bandhas*. Exhale, fold forward and deepen the *bandhas*. Bring your hands to the floor between your feet. Inhale, lengthen your spine, expand your chest and look forward. Exhale, fold back down into the posture and stay for five breaths. Inhale, lift your chest again, raising your gaze. Exhale, place your hands on your hips keeping your back long and flat. Inhale, come back up to standing. Exhale, stay with your hands on your hips ready for *Prasarita Padottanasana B*.

🏵 Nose

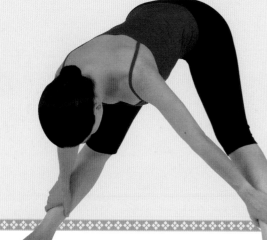

🌀 If you can't bring your hands to the floor comfortably, try taking your feet a little wider apart. If it is still difficult, then bend your legs a little. If you are still struggling, place your hands on your shins instead of the floor. Whichever modification you use, it is important to keep your back as flat as possible and fold from your hips rather than rounding your spine.

prasarita padottanasana B, C, D

From *Prasarita Padottanasana* A inhale and lift your chest. Exhale, fold forward deepening the *bandhas*. Stay here for five breaths. This is *Prasarita Padottanasana* B. Inhale, come back up to standing.

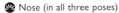 Nose (in all three poses)

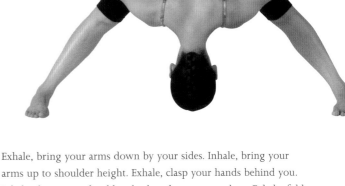

Exhale, bring your arms down by your sides. Inhale, bring your arms up to shoulder height. Exhale, clasp your hands behind you. Inhale, draw your shoulders back and open your chest. Exhale, fold forward, and bring your hands over your head. Stay here for five breaths. This is *Prasarita Padottanasana* C. Inhale, come back up to standing. Exhale, bring your arms down by your sides.

Inhale, bring your arms to shoulder height. Exhale, put your hands on your hips. Inhale, lift your chest. Exhale, fold forward and bring your hands to your feet, and hold your big toes with your first two fingers. Inhale, lift your chest. Exhale, draw your elbows toward the ceiling, your head toward the floor; shoulders stay broad. Stay for five breaths. This is *Prasarita Padottanasana* D. Inhale, lengthen your spine, open your chest, look forward. Exhale, hands on hips, back flat. Inhale, come back to standing. Exhale, step or jump your feet together at the front of your mat.

parsvottanasana

PARSVA = side; UTTANA = intense stretch; ASANA = posture

This deep standing forward bend helps to develop flexibility and lightness. Maintain a steady weight on both feet as you move into the pose, and breathe as fully as possible as you hold it.

Inhale, step or jump your feet apart, turning a quarter to your right to face the long side of your mat. Lift your arms to shoulder height. Exhale, turn your right foot out, left foot in. Face your right foot. Square your hips. Put your hands together in prayer position behind you. Inhale, expand your chest, roll your shoulders back and look up. Exhale, fold forward deeply with hips parallel. Stay for five breaths. Inhale, come up to standing and bring your feet parallel. Exhale, turn your feet to the left. Inhale, lift your chest. Exhale, fold forward over your leg. Stay for five breaths. Inhale, come up, turn your feet parallel, bring your arms to shoulder height. Exhale, step or jump your feet together to face the front of your mat. Bring your arms by your sides.

✿ Nose

☯ Take particular care to open the front surface of your body in this posture, and to keep your upper back and shoulders wide open by lifting your elbows slightly and keeping the back of your neck long and relaxed.

🌀 This pose deeply stretches the hamstring of your front leg. If it feels too intense, make the fold at your hips less deep – 90 degrees or less. Concentrate on keeping your hips parallel, your spine long and easy and the *bandhas* fully engaged. Avoid swaying the hip of your rear leg back, rounding your lower spine or hunching your shoulders. If you can't bring your hands to prayer pose behind your back, just hold your elbows with your hands instead.

utthita hasta padangusthasana A

UTTHITA = extended; HASTA = hand; PADANGUSTHA = big toe; ASANA = posture

This series of poses are a challenge in terms of balance, strength and flexibility. Make sure you don't sacrifice any one of these qualities for the others. Aim for a perfect synthesis of all three!

Inhale, bend your right knee and lift it toward your chest. Take hold of your right big toe with the first two fingers of your right hand. Bring your left hand to your left hip. Exhale, lift your right leg upward, stretching it out until it is fully straight. Draw your right shoulder back into line with the left. Stay for five breaths. Inhale. Exhale and go straight into the next pose: *Utthita Hasta Padangusthasana* B.

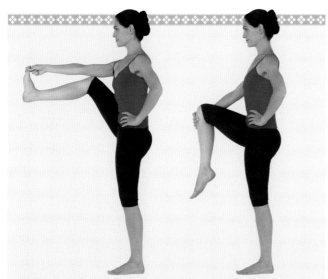

🌀 Creating a stable base that consists of your standing leg, abdominal muscles, low back and *bandhas* is more important than getting your lifted leg straight. So, if straightening your leg is difficult, take hold of your big toe and hold your lifted leg bent until your flexibility improves. Alternatively, keep your standing leg long and strong, draw your knee to your chest and hold it with your hand.

🌸 Toes

utthita hasta padangusthasana B

Exhale, open your right leg out to the side. Turn your head to look over your left shoulder. Press your right foot firmly away from you and your left foot down into the earth. Draw your right shoulder back toward the centre of your body to oppose the pull of your right foot. Keep the whole posture as strain-free as possible. Stay for five breaths. Inhale, draw your right leg back to the front and go straight into the next pose: *Utthita Hasta Padangusthasana* C.

❀ To the side

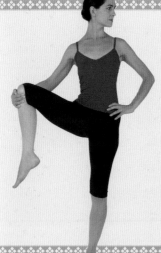

🌀 If you can't straighten your lifted leg in *Utthita Hasta Padangusthasana* A, keep it bent instead. Just draw your leg to the side and, holding your big toe, concentrate on opening out at the hip. If you were holding your knee with both hands in the previous pose, change your grip so that you hold your right knee with your right hand only. Put your left hand on your hip.

utthita hasta padangusthasana C, D

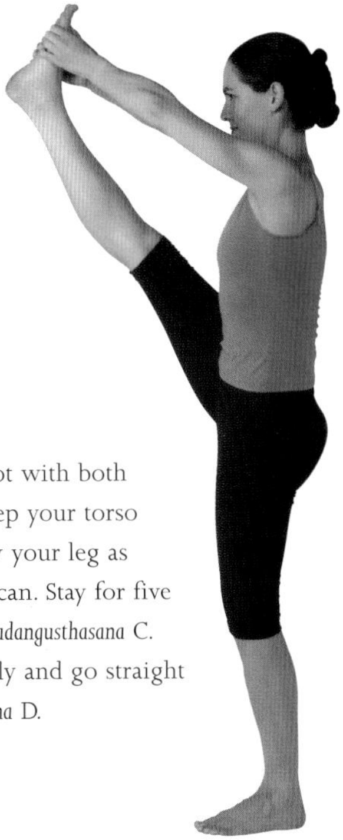

Exhale, take hold of your foot with both hands and lift it upward. Keep your torso completely vertical and draw your leg as tightly to your chest as you can. Stay for five breaths. This is *Utthita Hasta Padangusthasana* C. Inhale, lower your leg slightly and go straight into *Utthita Hasta Padangusthasana* D.

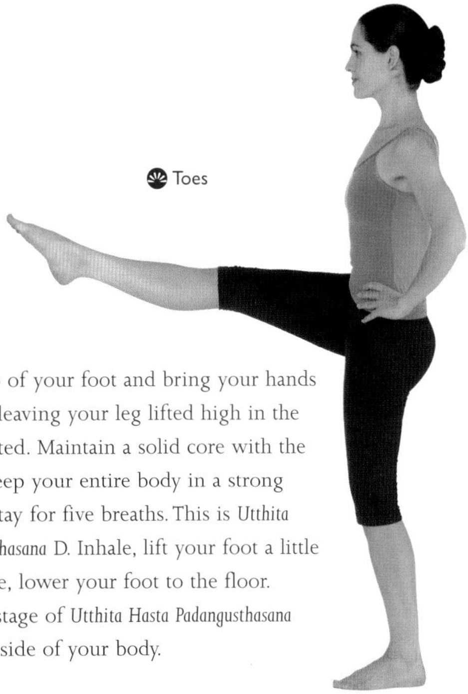

Exhale, let go of your foot and bring your hands to your hips leaving your leg lifted high in the air, toes pointed. Maintain a solid core with the *bandhas* and keep your entire body in a strong vertical lift. Stay for five breaths. This is *Utthita Hasta Padangusthasana* D. Inhale, lift your foot a little higher. Exhale, lower your foot to the floor. Repeat each stage of *Utthita Hasta Padangusthasana* on the other side of your body.

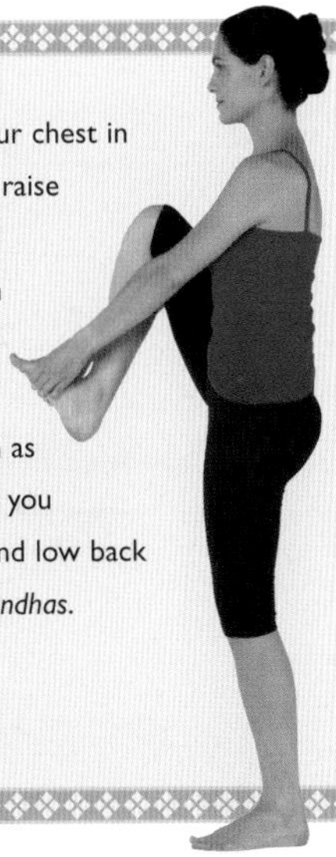

If you can't lift your leg to your chest in *Utthita Hasta Padangusthasana* C, raise your knee to your chest instead. Alternatively, hold your foot with both hands and lift your leg with your knee bent. Bring your thigh toward your chest as much as possible. Whichever modification you choose, keep your standing leg and low back straight and supported by the *bandhas*.

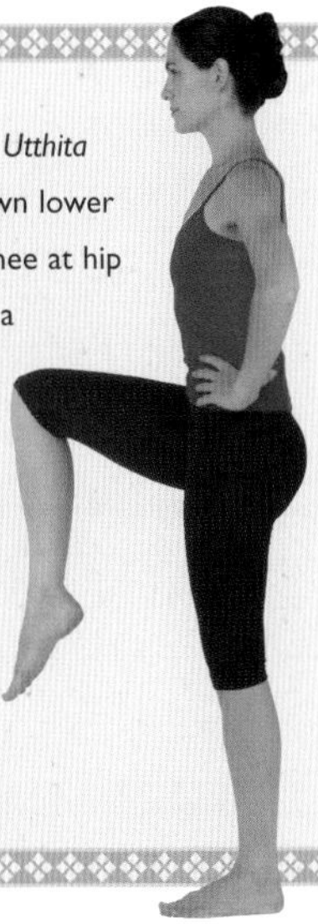

If you can't hold your leg high in *Utthita Hasta Padangusthasana* D, take it down lower or bend your knee and hold your knee at hip height. Make sure that you maintain a core of strength and stability in your standing leg, abdomen and low back. Don't let your chest sway back to act as a counterweight to your leg.

ardha baddha padmottanasana

ARDHA = half; BADDHA = bound; PADMA = lotus; UTTANA = intense stretch; ASANA = posture

The full pose has a nice gentle quality of surrender and ease, helping to develop an inner focus. If your hips are not yet very open, take the pose one step at a time and use a modification.

Inhale, lift your right foot and hold it with both hands. Exhale, fold your right foot into the top of your left thigh. Reach behind your back with your right hand to catch hold of your foot. Inhale, stretch your left arm up. Exhale, fold forward at your hips and place your left hand on the floor beside your foot. Inhale, lengthen your spine and look forward. Exhale, fold deeply toward your thigh. Stay for five breaths. Inhale, open your chest and look forward. Exhale, slightly bend your left knee to help you balance. Inhale, return to standing, taking your left arm over your head. Exhale, release your arms and legs back to standing. Repeat on the other side and go into the vinyasa shown.

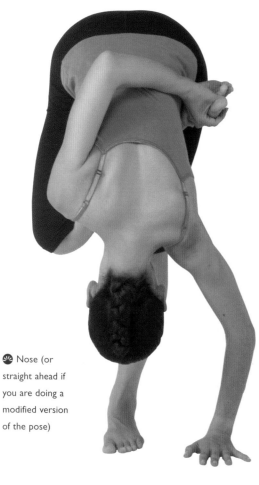

🪷 Nose (or straight ahead if you are doing a modified version of the pose)

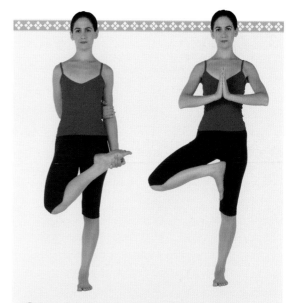

🪷 The sequence so far has not done a great deal to prepare you for this half-lotus position – avoid it if it causes discomfort in your knees. If you can't catch your foot with your hand behind your back, just hold it with your nearest hand. Alternatively, place your foot on your inner thigh and, instead of folding forward, stay standing for five breaths.

utkatasana

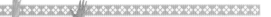

UTKA = fierce or mighty; ASANA = posture

Come into *Utkatasana* using the vinyasa shown in the above pictures.

From down-facing dog pose (see above) inhale and jump or step your feet between your hands. Bend your knees, drop your hips, keep the *bandhas* engaged, lift your torso and take your arms over your head, palms together. Feel a strong upward thrust of your body from your waist and a lengthening or downward movement in your hips. Stay here for five breaths. Move through a vinyasa (see pages 70–73) to come into the next pose: *Virabhadrasana* A.

❸ Keep your heels deeply rooted and the inner sides of your feet, ankles and knees together as you stretch. If you are weak in your abdominal and low back area, beware of pushing your hips too far back without any sense of weight in them. Use the combination of the *bandhas* and gravity to ground your pelvis and form a steady base from which to lift upward.

🌸 Thumbs

❹ If your shoulders feel hunched and tense when you put your palms together, try interlacing your fingers, holding your elbows or keeping your arms apart. This gives more breadth in your shoulders but allows you to maintain the upward thrust of your torso, the lengthening of your spine and the depth and fluidity of your breath.

virabhadrasana A

VIRABHADRA = warrior; ASANA = posture

From *Utkatasana* do the above vinyasa: exhale, fold forward. Inhale, lift your chest. Exhale into *Chaturanga*. Inhale into up-facing dog. Exhale into down-facing dog.

Inhale, turn your left heel in and step your right foot between your hands. Ground your back heel firmly into the floor. Raise your torso, take your arms over your head and bring your palms together. Look up at your thumbs. Stay for five deep breaths. Inhale, straighten your right leg, keep looking up and, maintaining the upward lift of your body, turn your feet to the other side. Exhale, bend your left knee in a deep lunge. Stay here for five breaths. Go straight into the next pose: *Virabhadrasana* B.

🌸 Thumbs

❸ The strong uplift of your arms in this position can draw your shoulder blades up, which allows you to bend your neck back to look up at your thumbs. In some Astanga yoga classes you may be taught the recent trend of drawing your shoulderblades back and down in upward looking poses. Although this produces an attractive posture, you should avoid it if it creates tension in your neck. Protect your low back from over-extension in this pose by contracting the *bandhas*. Cultivate a sense of dropping your tailbone downward as you lift your chest up.

virabhadrasana B

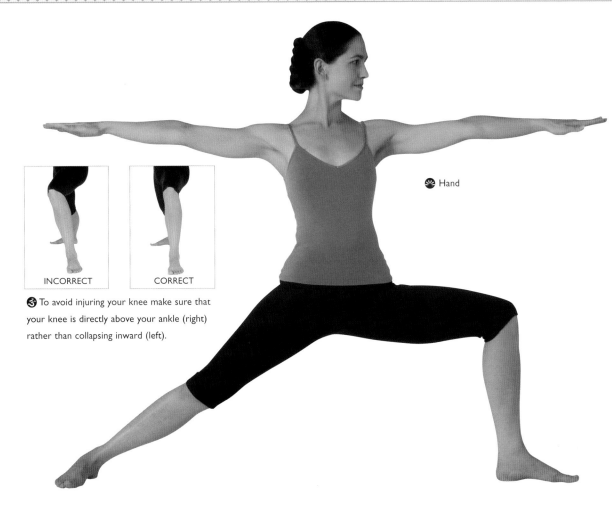

INCORRECT   CORRECT

🕉 To avoid injuring your knee make sure that your knee is directly above your ankle (right) rather than collapsing inward (left).

🌸 Hand

From *Virabhadrasana* A (see opposite) exhale, open your arms out to the sides, face the long edge of your mat and widen your stance. Maintain the deep bend in your left knee and ground the outer edge of your right foot firmly into the floor. Look over your left hand. Stay for five breaths. Inhale, straighten your left leg and turn your left foot inward. Exhale, turn your right foot outward and bend your right leg into a deep lunge, keeping your knee directly over your ankle. Stay for five breaths and then exhale, bringing your hands onto the floor on either side of your right foot. Go into the vinyasa in the pictures shown below: step back and lower your chest into *Chaturanga*. Inhale, move into up-facing dog. Exhale, move into down-facing dog.

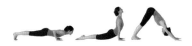

From down-facing dog jump or step through to *Dandasana*.

half vinyasa

This series of movements is performed after almost every posture of the Primary Series (the few exceptions are noted beside the relevant poses). They help to realign your spine, release any tension from the preceding posture and eliminate any potential negative effects – like a kind of slate-cleaning exercise. They also keep your whole body warm and active.

The true "full" vinyasa of Astanga Vinyasa yoga consists of a complete sun salutation but this is extremely demanding and few practitioners do it on a regular basis. What is known as a Half Vinyasa is shown on the opposite page. The movements should be repeated between each posture and on each side of an asymmetrical posture. They allow you to get to and from the basic seated position smoothly. The vinyasa are postures that you are already familiar with from the sun salutations (see pages 46–53) with the addition of a "jump back" and a "jump through" to sitting. The key to these jumps is the use of *mula* and *uddiyana bandhas* (see pages 35–36) – without them you will notice that you can hardly lift yourself from the floor!

The vinyasa

From sitting, cross your ankles and place your hands by your hips, fully engage the *bandhas* and press into your hands to lift yourself clear of the floor. Draw your legs back through your arms to jump into *Chaturanga*, continue through to up-facing dog, down-facing dog and then look toward the space between your hands. Bend your knees and jump your legs back through your arms (your hips have to go way up high here as if you were going to do a handstand) to come to sitting. Of course it is not quite that easy, but practice makes perfect and some modifications are possible; they are illustrated on the following pages.

Modifying the vinyasa

You can modify the vinyasa shown opposite by eliminating the jumping back and through. This frees you to concentrate on getting the *bandhas* working. Cross your legs, push your hands to the floor and lift the *bandhas* and yourself as high as you can. Roll forward bringing your hands and knees to the floor and step or jump back from there into a flat-back position. Now lower first your knees and then your chest to the floor, move your hands back a little and push up into up-facing dog and then back into down-facing dog. From here, step or hop your feet as far forward as you can with your ankles crossed and come to sitting. This is Modification A and is shown on page 72.

If you are just too exhausted to do this full range of movements every time then you can use Modification B on page 73 (top) in which you come to a crossed-legs position, push up lifting the *bandhas*, come back to sitting and then lift your arms overhead, lower them and go straight into the next pose. This does not work as well as the full thing but you may need to preserve some energy at first.

A further alternative is Modification C on page 73 (bottom). Here you omit the lift altogether and simply take your arms overhead and back down again. This helps to open your upper back and counterpose the huge number of forward bends but is much easier and may be useful when you are tired or need a softer practice.

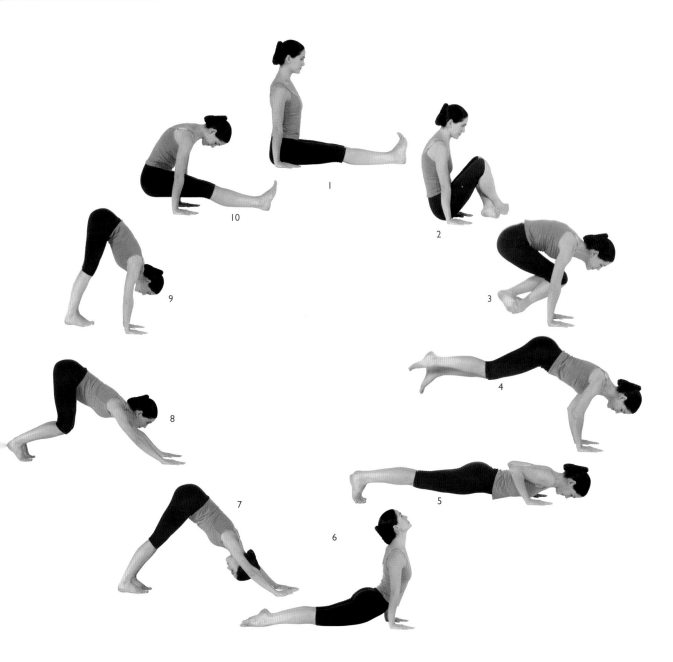

half vinyasa modifications

These three modified versions of the half vinyasa
shown on page 71 are a useful way of building up
your upper body strength. You can also
use a modification when you are tired
or want a softer practice.

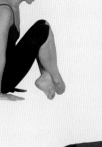

1

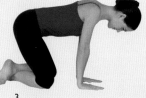

2

9

8

MODIFICATION A

3

4

7

6

5

MODIFICATION B

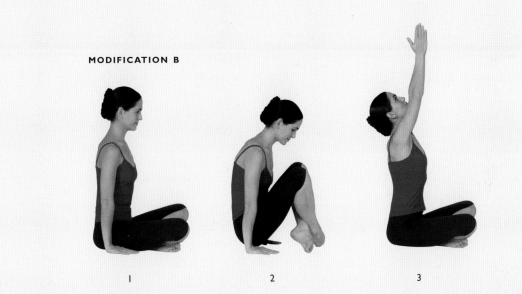

1   2   3

MODIFICATION C

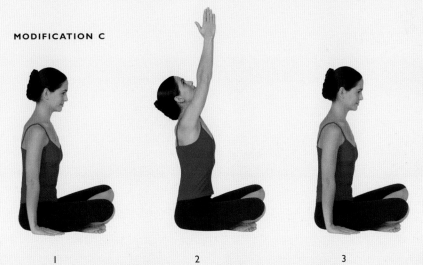

1   2   3

dandasana

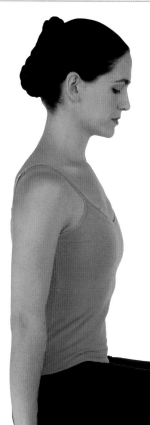

DANDA = stick; ASANA = posture

Despite its apparent simplicity, this pose demands your full attention and yields surprising results. A perfect balance of effort and relaxation is required to find equilibrium here, a great preparation for some of the more complicated poses to come.

Exhale, place your palms flat on the floor beside your hips. Push the soles of your feet firmly away from you, lengthening your legs and lifting your spine fully. Dip your chin toward your chest to create *jalandhara bandha* (see page 36). Keep your body active but not tense. Stay for five breaths. Go straight into the next pose: *Paschimottanansana*.

 Nose

🟣 If you can't sit upright with your legs straight, then let your knees bend a little. As in all yoga postures, the most important factor is the movement in your spine — your leg muscles will stretch over time.

paschimottanasana A, B, C

PASCHIMA = western; UTTANA = intense stretch; ASANA = posture

This is the seated version of *Padangusthasana* (see page 54). Gravity acts on the body in a different way now, but you can still apply much of the knowledge that you gained from the earlier pose here.

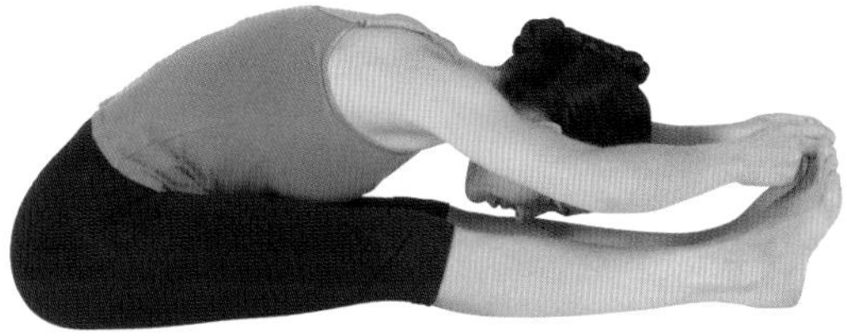

Exhale, fold forward at your hips with a long spine. Grasp your big toes with your first two fingers. Inhale, open your chest, lift your gaze and lengthen your spine. Exhale, fold forward, elbows to the sides. Stay for five breaths. Inhale, open your chest, lift your gaze and lengthen your spine. This is *Paschimottanasana* A. Go straight into the next pose.

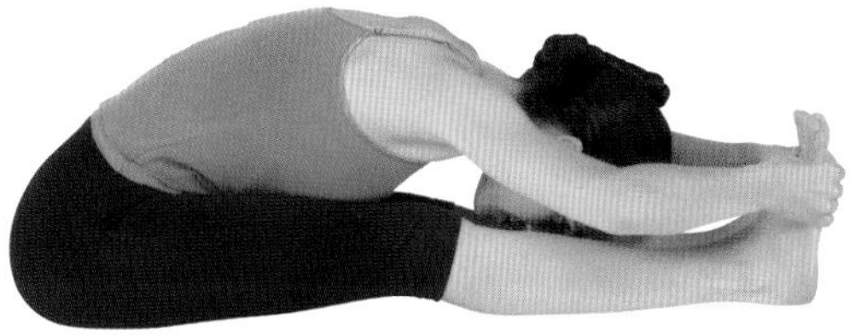

Exhale, hold the outer edges of your feet with your hands – thumbs on top of your feet. Inhale, open your chest, lift your gaze and lengthen your spine. Exhale, fold deeply forward at your hips and stay for five breaths. Inhale, open your chest, lift your gaze and lengthen your spine again. This is *Paschimottanasana* B. Go straight into the next pose.

Toes

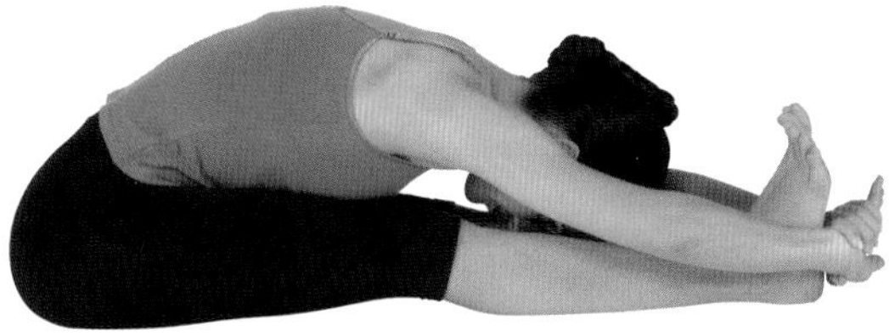

Exhale, stretch your wrists past your feet and clasp hold of one of your wrists with the other hand. Inhale, open your chest, lift your gaze and lengthen your spine. Exhale, fold forward deeply at your hips and stay for five breaths. Inhale, open your chest, lift your gaze and lengthen your spine again. This is *Paschimottanasana* C. Exhale, release your grasp and place your hands on the floor by your hips before going into a vinyasa.

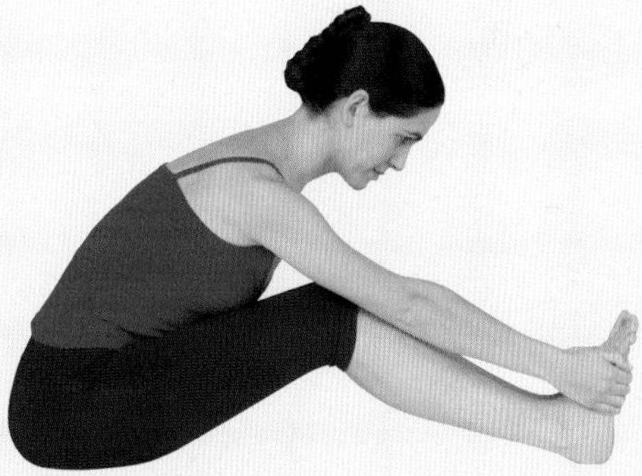

If you can't fold forward with your legs straight in any of these positions, bend your knees a little. Concentrate instead on lengthening your spine. If you can't hold your feet with your hands, hold your shins.

purvottanasana

PURVA = Eastern; UTTANA = intense stretch; ASANA = posture

This strong opening for the front surface of the body with backward rotated arms produces an interesting mixture of vulnerability and strength. Make sure that your shoulders sit directly above your wrists.

🔆 Nose

Exhale, bring your hands to the floor behind your back so that they are shoulder-width apart; fingers pointing toward your toes. Inhale, expand your chest, lift your hips up and release your head back. Press firmly into the floor with your feet, rolling your inner ankles, knees and thighs toward each other. Stay for five breaths. Exhale and lower your hips to the floor before going into a vinyasa.

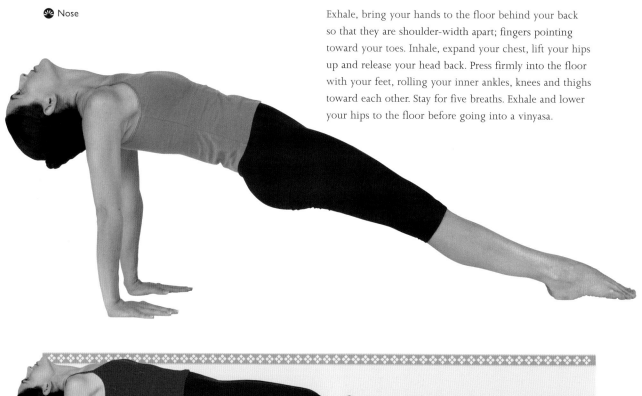

⊗ If you find it difficult to lift your whole body off the floor, do the pose with bent legs instead. This is easier and offers most of the same benefits as the full version of the pose. If your neck feels too tense when you tilt your head back, keep your chin on your chest.

ardha baddha padma paschimottanasana

ARDHA = half; BADDHA = bound; PADMA = lotus; PASCHIMA = western;

UTTANA = intense stretch; ASANA = posture

This is the sitting version of *Ardha Baddha Padmottanasana* (see page 66). The binding of the hand and foot here should produce a pleasant feeling of security and stability, not strain. Take great care of your bent knee.

Exhale, bend your right knee and hold your right foot with your left hand and your right knee with your right hand. Tuck your right foot as close in to your left hip as you can in a half-lotus position. Now take your right hand behind your back and catch hold of your right foot. Draw your knees toward each other slightly. Fold forward at your hips to bring your left hand to your left foot. Inhale, lift your chest and extend your spine. Exhale, fold as deeply forward as you can. Take five breaths. Inhale, lift your gaze and lengthen your spine. Exhale, release your foot, straighten your legs and go into a vinyasa. Repeat the pose on your left side and go into a vinyasa.

❁ Toes

🔴 Be careful that you don't damage your knees in this posture. If your hips are a little tight, the pose can transfer tension to your knee joint and strain it – so stop if you experience pain. If you find half-lotus difficult or uncomfortable, simply place your foot on the inside of your opposite thigh.

trianga mukhaikapada paschimottanasana

TRI = three; ANGA = limb; MUKHA = face; EKA = one; PADA = foot;
PASCHIMA = western; UTTANA = intense stretch; ASANA = posture

This is a valuable forward bend – although both legs face forwards at the hip, only one leg is stretched at the hamstring. This allows you to work each side individually with a very strong parallel hip position.

❋ Toes

Exhale, bend your right knee so your right foot is by your right hip with the sole facing up and your knees close together. Fold forward and grasp your left foot. Draw your spine long and keep folding deeply at your hip. Inhale, open your chest and lift your gaze. Exhale and fold forward again. Stay for five breaths. Inhale, open your chest and lengthen your spine. Exhale, straighten both legs. Go into a vinyasa. Repeat the pose on the other side and go into a vinyasa.

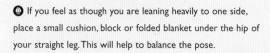

ⓘ If you feel as though you are leaning heavily to one side, place a small cushion, block or folded blanket under the hip of your straight leg. This will help to balance the pose.

ⓘ If your ankle or top of your foot is under too much pressure in a bent leg position, place a rolled-up blanket or small pad under your ankle for support. If the posture hurts your knee, do *Janu Sirsasana* (see pages 79–81) instead.

janu sirsasana A

JANU = knee; SIRSA = head; ASANA = posture

In this seated forward bend imagine that you are pushing your torso toward your extended leg using the muscles of your middle/lower back, rather than pulling with your arms and shoulders.

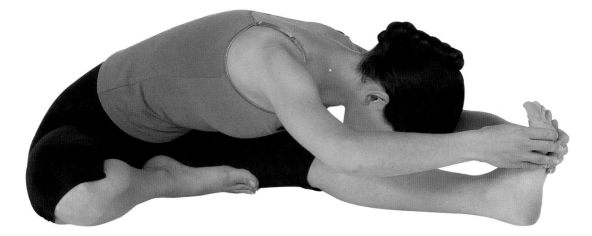

Exhale, bend your right knee and bring the sole of your foot into your left inner thigh. There should be a 90 degree angle between your bent knee and your straight leg. Fold forward at your hips bringing your hands to your left foot. Inhale, lift and open your chest. Exhale, fold deeply forward and hold the pose for five breaths. Inhale, lift your chest and raise your gaze. Exhale, release your foot, straighten both legs and go into a vinyasa. Repeat the pose on your left side. Go into a vinyasa.

🌀 Toes

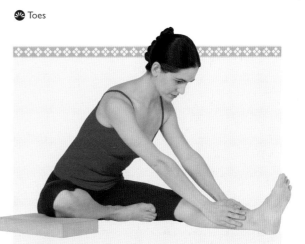

⏰ If your bent knee is a long way off the floor, support it using a cushion or rolled-up blanket. If you can't reach your foot with your hands, hold onto your shin instead.

🌀 This posture involves a deep but delicate twist in your low abdominal area. Take particular care to monitor *uddiyana bandha* (see page 36) as you exhale and fold forward.

janu sirsasana B

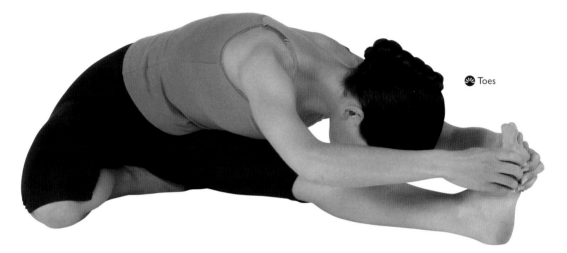

🌸 Toes

Come to a seated position as for *Janu Sirsasana* A. Exhale, place your hands behind you and lift your hips up and forward to sit your perineum over the heel of your right foot. The top of your foot rests on the floor and the angle between your knees is slightly less than in *Janu Sirsasana* A. Reach forward and hold your left foot with your hands.

Inhale, lengthen and open your chest. Exhale, fold forward deeply at your hips drawing your chest toward your shin. Stay for five breaths. Inhale, lift your chest and raise your gaze. Exhale, release the posture and stretch out both legs before going into a vinyasa. Repeat on the left side. Go into a vinyasa.

🌀 If you can't reach your left foot, hold your shin instead. If you can't comfortably rest the weight of your body on the top of your heel, either take the pressure off by putting your hands on the floor by your sides or simply repeat *Janu Sirsasana* A. Alternatively, just leave this posture out for the time being. Don't force your knees and ankles into this position — go slowly and carefully.

janu sirsasana C

🌀 Flex and turn out your foot so that the ball of your foot faces the floor. Lift your heel to a vertical position.

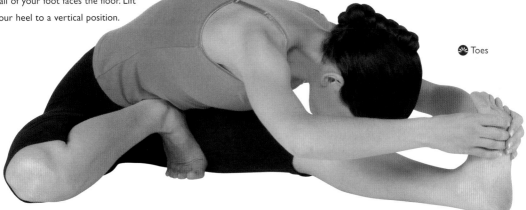

🌸 Toes

Exhale, bend your right knee, hold the heel of your right foot in your left hand and your toes in your right hand. Bring your foot to the inner thigh of your left leg (see inset picture). Bring your knees closer together than in *Janu Sirsasana* B. Reach forward and grasp your left foot. Inhale, open your chest,

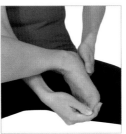

lengthen your spine and lift your gaze. Exhale, fold forward keeping your chest broad. Stay for five breaths. Inhale, lift your chest and lengthen your spine. Exhale, stretch out both legs before going into a vinyasa. Repeat on the left side. Go into a vinyasa.

🔵 If you are reasonably close to doing this pose, a block or cushion placed under your hips may give you the help you need to complete the pose. If, however, you can't make the huge rotation at the knee that the pose demands, then stay in the preparatory position with your hands holding your foot, or repeat *Janu Sirsasana* A. Alternatively, just leave this posture out for the time being.

marichyasana A

MARICHI = the name of a sage; ASANA = posture
The four variations of this posture all have a beneficial effect on your digestive system.

✺ Toes

Exhale, bend your right leg and bring your right foot to the floor directly opposite your right hip. Bend forward and extend your right arm on the inside of your right knee toward your left toes. Wrap your right arm around your knee keeping your armpit low on your shin. Take your left arm around your back and grasp your left wrist with your right hand. Inhale, lift your chest and lengthen your spine. Exhale, fold fully into the pose and stay for five breaths. Inhale, lift your chest and lengthen your spine. Exhale, release and stretch both legs out before going into a vinyasa. Repeat on the other side. Go into a vinyasa.

🕉 If you can't clasp your hands behind your back, place your hands on the floor and bring your chest as far forward past your knee as possible. If you can nearly clasp your hands, use a belt, strap or sock to help bridge the gap.

marichyasana B

Exhale, bring your left leg into half-lotus. Bend your right knee and bring your right foot to the floor in line with your right sitting bone. Lean forward – your left heel should press into your lower abdomen – and reach your right arm forward and wrap it around your leg. Take your left arm around your back to meet your right and clasp your left wrist with your right hand. Inhale, lengthen your spine and look forward. Exhale, fold into a deep forward bend. Stay for five breaths. Inhale, raise your head and lengthen your spine. Exhale, release the pose and stretch both legs out before going into a vinyasa. Repeat on the other side. Go into a vinyasa.

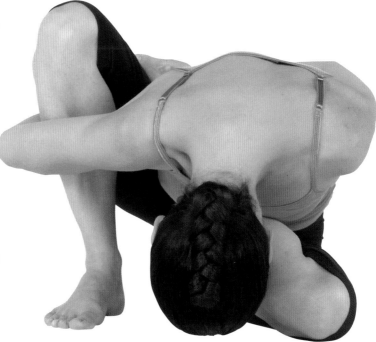

🌀 Nose

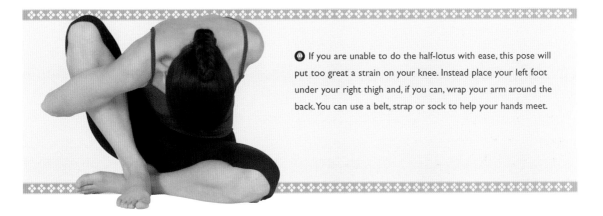

🌀 If you are unable to do the half-lotus with ease, this pose will put too great a strain on your knee. Instead place your left foot under your right thigh and, if you can, wrap your arm around the back. You can use a belt, strap or sock to help your hands meet.

marichyasana C

Exhale, bend your right leg bringing your foot close to your right hip, opposite the sitting bone. Rotate your torso toward your right knee until you can bring your left arm across the front of your knee. Turn the palm of your hand to face backward and wrap your arm around your knee. Bring your right arm around your back and clasp your right wrist with your left hand. Your left foot presses open and forward. Inhale, lengthen your spine and create a strong vertical lift. Exhale, turn to look over your right shoulder and stay for five breaths. Inhale, look to the front. Exhale, release the pose and stretch both legs out before going into a vinyasa. Repeat on the other side. Go into a vinyasa.

☀ Over your shoulder

The arm position in *Marichyasana C* requires a huge amount of shoulder flexibility as well as twisting in your spine. If it is too difficult, simply hold your right knee with your left hand and place your right hand on the floor to help to steady and lift your spine. Don't slump and let all your weight rest on your right hand though.

marichyasana D

Exhale, bring your left foot into half-lotus. Bend your right knee and place your foot in line with your sitting bone. Bring your left knee as close to your right foot as you can. Rotate your torso and stretch your left arm along the outside of your right knee. Turn your palm to face backward and wrap your arm around your knee, taking your right arm behind your back. Clasp your right wrist with your left hand. Inhale, lengthen your spine and look over your right shoulder. Exhale, deepen the twist. Stay for five breaths. Inhale, turn your head to the front. Exhale, release the pose and stretch both legs out before going into a vinyasa. Repeat on the other side. Go into a vinyasa.

🅰 Over your shoulder

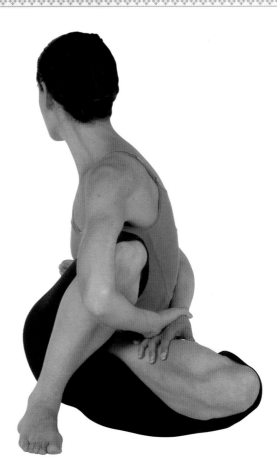

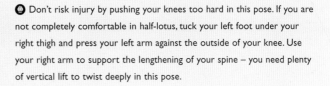

🅰 Don't risk injury by pushing your knees too hard in this pose. If you are not completely comfortable in half-lotus, tuck your left foot under your right thigh and press your left arm against the outside of your knee. Use your right arm to support the lengthening of your spine – you need plenty of vertical lift to twist deeply in this pose.

navasana

NAVA = boat; ASANA = posture

This is the only pose that is repeated five times in the Primary Series. It is a test of strength and endurance, but also a balancing pose, that needs lightness and ease.

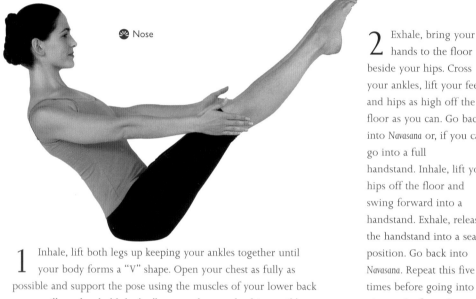

✿ Nose

1 Inhale, lift both legs up keeping your ankles together until your body forms a "V" shape. Open your chest as fully as possible and support the pose using the muscles of your lower back – you will need to hold the *bandhas* strongly to make this possible. Bring your arms straight out in front of you on either sides of your legs, parallel to the floor and palms facing. Stay for five breaths.

2 Exhale, bring your hands to the floor beside your hips. Cross your ankles, lift your feet and hips as high off the floor as you can. Go back into *Navasana* or, if you can, go into a full handstand. Inhale, lift your hips off the floor and swing forward into a handstand. Exhale, release the handstand into a seated position. Go back into *Navasana*. Repeat this five times before going into a vinyasa (as far as down-facing dog). Go straight into the next pose: *Bhujapidasana*

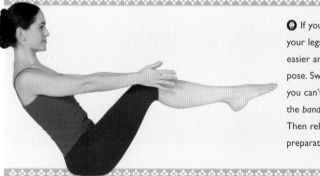

● If you don't have the strength or flexibility to straighten your legs in *Navasana*, do the pose with bent legs. This is much easier and will strengthen your body in preparation for the full pose. Swinging into a handstand from *Navasana* is difficult – if you can't do it, simply press your hands into the floor, engage the *bandhas* deeply, and lift your hips and feet just off the floor. Then release and go back into *Navasana*. This is good preparatory work for the handstand.

bhujapidasana

BHUJA = arm; PIDA = pressure; ASANA = posture
As with the previous pose, this one requires just as much finesse in terms of balance and control as it does muscle strength.

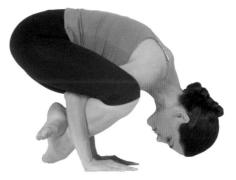

1 From down-facing dog inhale and jump forward bringing your legs around the outsides of your arms. Cross your ankles. Now slowly draw your feet backward and your head forward until you can balance with both your feet and forehead just off the floor. Stay for five breaths.

🪷 Nose

2 Inhale, uncross your ankles, release your legs and go into *Tittibhasana* (this is a transitional pose). Exhale, jump back to *Chaturanga* (see page 46). Go into a vinyasa (as far as down-facing dog) and then straight into the next pose: *Kurmasana*.

🌀 Jumping into *Bhujapidasana* requires strength and practice. Instead, jump your feet forward to land on the floor on either side of your hands. Then sit back on your arms and cross your ankles. Keep your forearms vertical, elbows above wrists. Hovering above the floor is also difficult – you may want to rest your head gently on the floor. On the way out of the pose it may be easier to jump back than it was to jump forward. If not, drop your feet to the floor and then step or jump back.

kurmasana

KURMA = tortoise; ASANA = posture

Approach this pose slowly and steadily as if you have all the time in the world – much like a tortoise!
If you can't do the pose straight away, aim to ease into it day by day.

From down-facing dog, inhale and jump your feet forward so that your legs land on your upper arms in *Tittibhasana* (see page 87). Lower your hips to the floor and release your chest forward, threading your arms under your legs until your knees are near your shoulders. Lengthen your body as much as possible, rolling your pubic bone toward the floor and broadening your chest with your arms and legs outstretched. Stay for five breaths. Go straight into the next posture: *Supta Kurmasana*.

🌓 Third eye

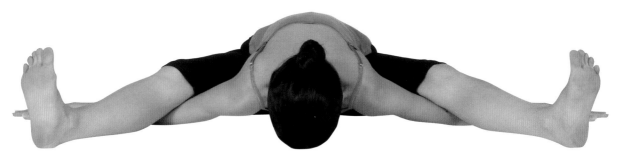

⚙ If you can't jump your legs into *Tittibhasana*, jump your feet to the outer sides of your hands and then lower your hips to the floor. If your shoulders won't slip easily under your arms, place your feet on the floor a little wider than chest-width apart and fold forward at your hips with a long straight spine. Place your hands on your knees or shins and draw your chest toward the floor (see left). If this is easy, thread your arms under your knees and rest your hands on the floor (see right) or reach round to hold your ankles. Draw your chest closer to the floor in this way.

supta kurmasana

SUPTA = sleeping; KURMA = tortoise; ASANA = posture

This is an intense pose that may take you many years to perfect. I am unable to perform the full posture, where the legs cross over the back of the neck, so the picture below shows a modification.

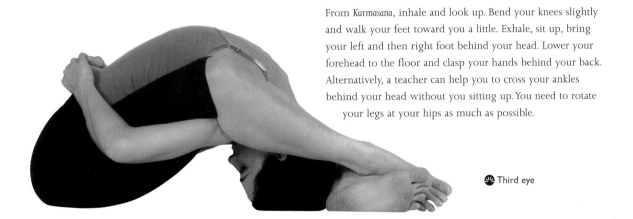

From *Kurmasana*, inhale and look up. Bend your knees slightly and walk your feet toward you a little. Exhale, sit up, bring your left and then right foot behind your head. Lower your forehead to the floor and clasp your hands behind your back. Alternatively, a teacher can help you to cross your ankles behind your head without you sitting up. You need to rotate your legs at your hips as much as possible.

🌑 Third eye

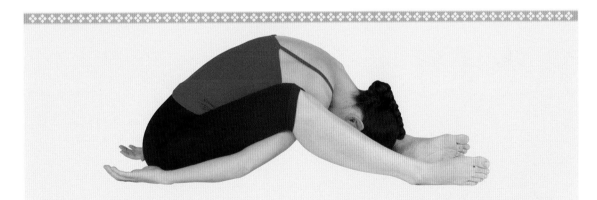

🌑 If you find *Kurmasana* very difficult leave *Supta Kurmasana* out. Alternatively, you can try this modification: from *Kurmasana*, draw your feet toward each other and cross your ankles – or bring the soles of your feet together – on the floor in front of you. Stay for five breaths, inhale and then lift back up to *Tittibhasana* (see page 87), bend your knees while balancing on your arms (this posture is called *Bakasana*) and jump back. Alternatively, release your legs and roll forward to place your hands on the floor, then step or jump your feet back before going into a vinyasa.

garbha pindasana

GARBHA = womb; PINDA = embryo; ASANA = posture

This tightly knotted pose is challenging but fun. With practice the rocking movement becomes a controlled, precise and delicate manoeuvre.

🌸 Nose

Exhale, come into lotus position, right leg first, then left. Slide your arms through the legs, bend your elbows and hold your face cupped in your hands. Inhale, lengthen your spine and take five breaths. Exhale, tuck your head into your hands and roll backward as you exhale and forward as you inhale. Do this nine times and rotate a complete clockwise circle in the process. Inhale, come back up to the front and go straight into the next pose: *Kukkutasana*.

🌀 The nine rocking motions in this pose symbolize the nine months of gestation.

🧘 If you can't do a full lotus, do half lotus and hold your arms around your legs. Alternatively, cross your legs and hold your ankles with your arms around your legs.

kukkutasana

KUKKUTA = cockerel; ASANA = posture

The pressure on your liver and spleen in this pose has a cleansing effect on the body.

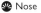 Nose

From *Garbha Pindasana*, inhale and roll forward onto your hands. Balance in this position for five breaths. Exhale, release the pose and stretch out your legs before going into a vinyasa.

If you used a half-lotus or a crossed-leg position in the last pose, you will need to do a lot of strong work with the *bandhas* to help you lift your legs and body off the floor. It is difficult but not impossible!

baddha konasana A

BADDHA = bound; KONA = angle; ASANA = posture

The term *baddha* (bound) refers to the clasping of your feet. This creates a circuit of energy in your body. Hold your feet firmly but tenderly – don't grip them like a vice!

Exhale, bring the soles of your feet together and let your knees relax to the sides. Hold your feet with your hands so that your thumbs are on the soles and your fingers are on the tops of your feet. Open your feet outward like a book. Draw your spine long and lower your chin toward your throat. Stay for five breaths. Inhale and look forward. Go straight into the next pose: *Baddha Konasana B.*

🌀 Nose

🌀 If you find this pose difficult, it may help to lift your hips a little by sitting on a yoga block. If you can't reach your feet without rounding your back, then hold your shins instead. You should be aiming for the maximum lift in your spine, so direct most of your attention to achieving this, and don't worry too much about where your knees are – they will drop lower in time.

baddha konasana B

From *Baddha Konasana* A, exhale and fold forward bringing your chest and chin down toward the floor while keeping your back flat. Stay for five breaths. Inhale, lift up to sitting and look forward. Exhale, round your back and draw your head toward your feet making a deep curve in your spine. Hold for five breaths. Inhale, sit up, lift your spine and look forward. Exhale and stretch out your legs before going into a vinyasa.

🌸 Nose

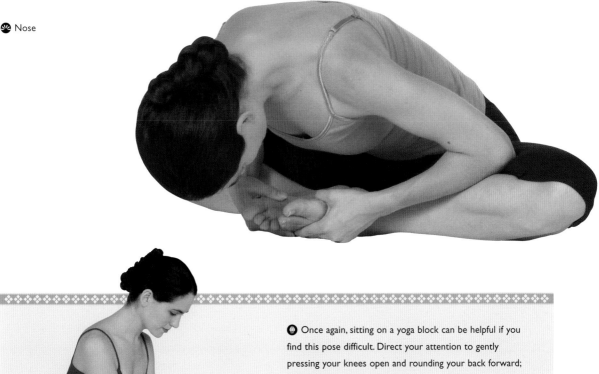

🌀 Once again, sitting on a yoga block can be helpful if you find this pose difficult. Direct your attention to gently pressing your knees open and rounding your back forward; folding forward with a flat back will come with time and practice. Make sure that you fully engage your low abdominal muscles to help support your spine.

upavishta konasana A and B

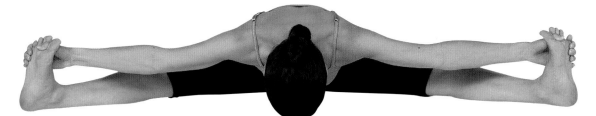

UPAVISHTA = seated; KONA = angle; ASANA = posture

The lift and strength of your lower back are important in these two poses.

Don't spread your legs out so widely that you lose the abdominal support for your spine.

Exhale, take your feet wide apart with your legs straight and your knees facing upward (they have a tendency to roll inward). Fold forward with your spine long and straight. Hold onto the outside edges of your feet with your hands. Inhale, lift your chest, look forward and lengthen your spine. Exhale, fold forward as deeply as possible and hold this position for five breaths. This is *Upavishta Konasana* A. Inhale, lift into the next pose: *Upavishta Konasana* B.

🌸 Third eye

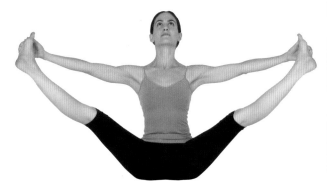

Expand your chest and broaden your shoulders. Use the *bandhas* for support. Stay for five breaths. Exhale, let go of your feet, cross your ankles and bring your palms to the floor before going into a vinyasa.

⚙ If you can't reach your feet in *Upavishta Konasana* A, hold onto your ankles or shins. If you find it difficult to straighten your legs in *Upavishta Konasana* B, hold your toes with your knees bent. Work on developing your balance and *bandha* control until your hamstrings loosen. If you can't lift straight up into *Upavishta Konasana* B, sit upright with your arms extended outwards and lift your legs to meet your hands.

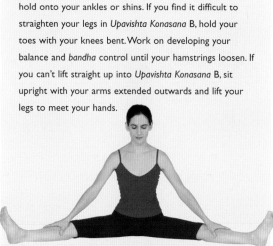

supta konasana

SUPTA = sleeping; KONA = angle; ASANA = posture

This wonderful pose must be one that every child has tried spontaneously. As an adult you may need encouragement to attempt the drop forward – it can seem a long way down!

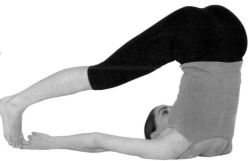

1 Exhale, roll back onto your shoulders taking your legs wide apart. Catch hold of your big toes with the first two fingers of each hand. Straighten your legs and stay for five breaths.

✦ Nose

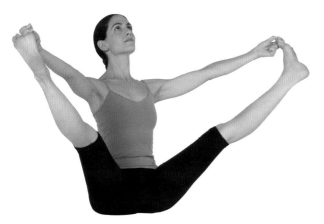

2 Inhale, roll upright to balance on your sitting bones in a wide upward-facing "V" shape (as for *Upavishta Konasana B*).

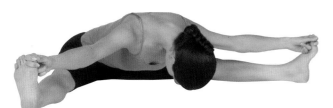

3 Exhale, drop forward to the floor with straight legs. Concentrate as you do this – the body's reflex action is to bend the knees just before impact and you need to override this. Make sure that the backs of your calves land before your heels to cushion the landing. Inhale, lift your chest and look ahead. Exhale and release your feet before going into a vinyasa.

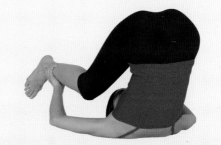

⊙ If you can't hold your toes with your legs straight, keep them bent or hold onto your ankles or shins instead. Until your legs are more flexible, concentrate on breathing deeply during the balance with your chest fully lifted. If you do the pose with bent legs, omit the forward drop which would hurt your heels. Instead release your legs from your hands and lower them slowly and gently.

supta padangusthasana A

SUPTA = sleeping; PADA = foot; ANGUSTHA = big toe; ASANA = posture

These are the reclining versions of the standing balances on pages 63–65. Because you don't need to balance here, you can focus on extending your legs and stabilizing your torso with the *bandhas*.

Exhale, lie on your back. Inhale, lift your right leg and take hold of your big toe with the first two fingers of your right hand. Place your left hand as far down your left thigh as you can reach. Keep both legs strong and straight with the balls of your feet open. Exhale, engage the *bandhas* and lift your head and chest off the floor bringing your forehead toward your right shin. Keep your left arm stretching strongly down your left leg. Inhale, release your head and shoulders back down to the floor (your legs stay straight) and go straight into the next pose: *Supta Padangusthasana B*.

✿ Toes

☸ This pose and the two that follow are the lying-down equivalents of the standing postures *Utthita Hasta Padangusthasana*. Here your body is supported by the floor and you don't have to balance, which means you can concentrate on stretching. This will enhance your ability to do *Utthita Hasta Padangusthasana*.

⊕ If you can't hold your big toe with your leg straight, bend your leg, hold your ankle or loop a belt over your foot instead. Don't forget to keep the leg on the floor grounded and your low abdominal muscles fully active in this pose.

supta padangusthasana B and C

❀ To the side

From *Supta Padangusthasana* A, exhale, keep hold of your big toe and lower your right leg to the floor on your right side. Turn your head to look over your left shoulder. Keep your left leg long and grounded, left hand on your left thigh. This is *Supta Padangusthasana* B. Stay for five breaths. Inhale, bring your right leg back up to centre and go straight into the next pose: *Supta Padangusthasana* C.

🌀 If you can't hold your toe with your leg straight in *Supta Padangusthasana* A, then in B you need to lower your leg to the floor with your knee bent. If you are using a strap, lower your leg as far to the floor as you can without your left hip lifting off the floor.

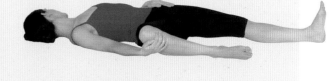

❀ Toes

Exhale, hold your right foot, keeping your head and shoulders on the floor. Keep your left leg strong and active. Press the ball of your left foot away from you. Draw your right leg toward your body, chest and shoulders as relaxed as possible. This is *Supta Padangusthasana* C. Stay for five breaths. Inhale, relax your left leg. Exhale, lower your right leg to the floor. Now repeat each pose on the other side and go into the vinyasa on the next page: *Chakrasana*.

🌀 If you can't hold your foot with both hands, hold your leg instead. Alternatively, bring your leg into your chest with your knee bent – this is useful if you are stiff in your lower back or hamstrings because it helps to open these areas.

chakrasana

CHAKRA = wheel; ASANA = posture

This backward roll lets you flow seamlessly from your back into a seated posture. It keeps the energy and pace of the practice and, once mastered is a pleasingly neat and economical move.

Lie on your back, bend your knees, bring your feet close to your hips and rest your hands on the floor behind your shoulders so that your fingers are pointing toward your body. Swing your knees toward your chest, lift your hips from the floor so that your feet go over your head toward the floor behind you. Keep your head completely square at all stages – resist the temptation to turn your head to the side as this can cause neck injury. Push very firmly down into the floor with your hands as your legs move over your head and start to straighten your arms. This takes the weight off the back of your head and allows your spine to uncurl completely. Let your feet come to the floor in a very narrow down-facing dog. Spring your hands forward into *Chaturanga* (see page 46) and then continue the vinyasa with up-facing dog and down-facing dog, then jump through to sitting.

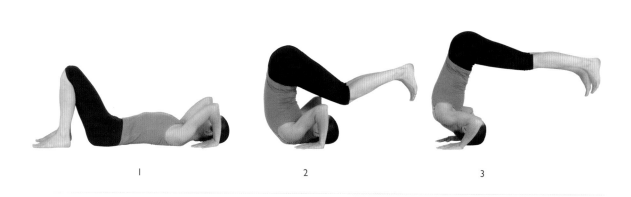

1   2   3

🔆 *Chakrasana* is a special kind of vinyasa that occurs in the primary series on three occasions when you finish a posture on your back. Some people also do *Chakrasana* after *Urdhva Dhanurasana* (see page 104). A graceful and logical way of returning to an upright position, *Chakrasana* consists of a backward roll followed by a jump back into *Chaturanga* position – from here you can continue in an ordinary vinyasa. It is not possible to learn *Chakrasana* safely from a book – you should seek a good teacher to help you master this move.

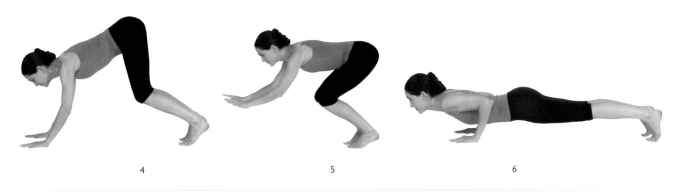

4   5   6

Although there aren't any modifications for this pose, a teacher can assist you by lifting you into *Chakrasana* – this is a great way to gain confidence. If you don't have access to a teacher or you have any concerns about your neck, don't attempt *Chakrasana*. Instead, sit up and do your usual form of vinyasa.

ubhaya padangusthasana

UBHAYA = both; PADA = foot; ANGUSTHA = big toe; ASANA = posture

This posture is fun to experiment with and lightens the heart. Keep your chest wide and your shoulders broad. If you let your shoulders collapse in toward your chest, you will roll over backward again!

🌼 Nose

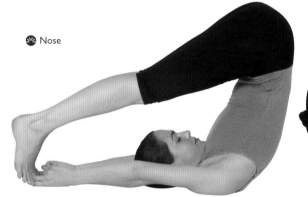

1 Exhale, roll backward and bring your feet onto the floor behind you. Keep your ankles together and clasp your big toes with the first two fingers of each hand.

2 Inhale, roll up to balance in an upward-facing "V" shape. Open your chest and draw your shoulders wide. Stay for five breaths. Exhale, release your legs and bring your feet softly to the floor before going into a vinyasa.

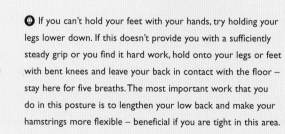

🔵 If you can't hold your feet with your hands, try holding your legs lower down. If this doesn't provide you with a sufficiently steady grip or you find it hard work, hold onto your legs or feet with bent knees and leave your back in contact with the floor – stay here for five breaths. The most important work that you do in this posture is to lengthen your low back and make your hamstrings more flexible – beneficial if you are tight in this area.

urdhva mukha paschimottanasana

URDHVA = upward; MUKHA = face; PASCHIMA = western; UTTANA = stretch; ASANA = posture

If you experience neck tension when you look toward your toes in this posture, drop your gaze a little lower. Direct your attention to your toes mentally instead.

❀ Toes

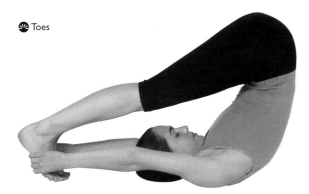

1 Exhale, roll backward to take hold of your feet, as in *Ubhaya Padangusthasana*, but this time hold onto the outside edges of your feet with your hands.

2 Inhale, roll up to a balancing position, pointing your toes and bringing your legs and chest as close together as possible. Stay for five breaths. Exhale, release the pose and bring your feet down to the floor before going into a vinyasa.

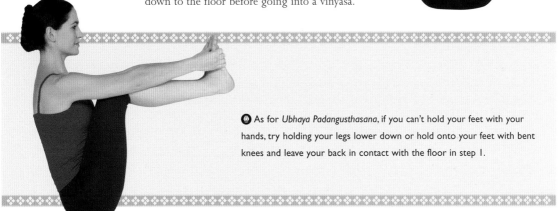

⊕ As for *Ubhaya Padangusthasana*, if you can't hold your feet with your hands, try holding your legs lower down or hold onto your feet with bent knees and leave your back in contact with the floor in step 1.

setu bandhasana

SETU = bridge; BANDHA = binding or contraction; ASANA = posture

This backbend, which acts as a counterpose to the previous poses, strengthens your legs, neck and back. It is worse in anticipation than in reality! Use a modification if you don't feel ready to try it yet.

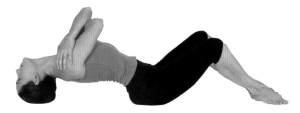 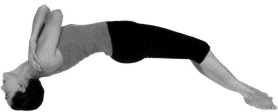

1 Lie on your back with knees bent. Exhale, turn your feet outward until the sides contact the floor and your heels are touching. Relax your knees toward the floor. Bring your arms by your body, palms down. Press your hands into the floor and arch your back by lifting your chest. Roll your head back to balance on your crown, hips, forearms and feet. Cross your arms and put your hands on your shoulders.

❸ This pose demands real strength and stability in your neck, and the confidence to move into it fully using your breath. In its full form it gives a strong opening to your chest and, once you have

2 Inhale, push with your feet to bring your hips off the floor. This enables you to roll on to the top of your head and perhaps your forehead. Keep your arms across your chest with hands on opposite shoulders. Stay for five breaths. Exhale, roll down from the posture, then go through *chakrasana*, vinyasa and back through to sitting.

❀ Nose

your balance, the pose feels remarkably secure. It is best learned under the guidance of a teacher who will check your technique and give you confidence.

---

❶ If you have any weakness or injury in your neck or shoulders, it is advisable to use a modification. Try doing the posture with your hands supporting the backs of your hips and

your elbows on the floor. Or simply go as far as step one but instead of crossing your arms over your chest, leave them resting on the floor alongside your body.

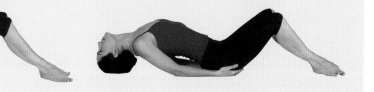

the finishing sequence

The last 14 postures of the sequence are designed to rebalance and restore the fine tuning of the body and mind after the rigorous practice of the Primary Series.

The finishing sequence includes a series of deep backbends, seated and inverted postures. The shoulderstand and the postures that follow have a pacifying effect. They quieten the breath and the heart, and turn the mind inward. The headstand is a test of balance and calm that requires focus and control without tension; a kind of elegant, effortless stability. The peaceful equilibrium of *Padmasana*, the lotus position, is followed with one final hurdle: *Tolasana*, the scales posture.

Tolasana demands that you dig down deep for your last resources of strength and endurance. It is supposed to be held for 100 fairly rapid breaths, something that should be worked up to over time. Its position as the penultimate posture of the series makes it the final peak in a long upward climb. It is followed by the bliss of the simple resting pose, *Savasana*. The extraordinary contrast between these two postures is a profound experience. Like diving from the heat of the sun into cool water, the two postures represent the poles of physical sensation, from the concentrated power needed to lift yourself off the earth into the utter stillness of total rest.

However much of the Primary Series you practise, you will need to include at least some elements, if not all, of the finishing sequence to complete your practice. If you need to do a shorter or modified form of the Primary Series, have a look at the sequences on pages 118–121 to give you some ideas. The very minimum that you should do is close with *Savasana*, which is the vital restorative and digestive phase of finishing sequence. Tempting though it may be to jump up and get on with your day, full of the energy the practice creates, make sure you leave time for *Savasana*. The posture completes the cycle, allowing for assimilation of the practice at a deep level and a restoration of the equilibrium needed for everyday living.

urdhva dhanurasana

URDHVA = upward; DHANURA = bow; ASANA = posture

The posture should open the front surface of your spine, not just hinge in your lower back. If it hurts, stop and do a modification.

1 Exhale, lie on your back and bend your knees with your feet hip-width apart and parallel. Bring your hands flat on the floor above your shoulders, fingers pointing to your shoulders, elbows lifting straight upward. Inhale, lift your hips off the floor.

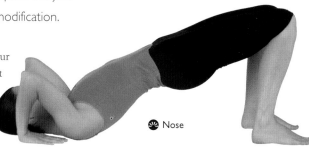

❀ Nose

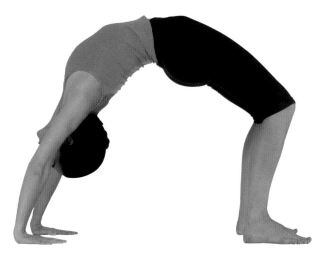

2 Push deeply into your hands and feet to take your head and shoulders into a full backbend. Stay for five breaths. Exhale, come down. Repeat twice more. Inhale, return to sitting. Exhale, fold forward into *Paschimottanasana* A (see page 75) for five breaths. Inhale, lift and lengthen your spine, look forward. Exhale and release before going into a vinyasa.

❸ This backbend is less about great strength and more about a huge opening and stretching of your chest. You can secure the posture by keeping your big toes and thumbs firmly rooted to the floor. Although letting them lift may create the sensation of more "space", it produces an unstable posture that stresses your joints.

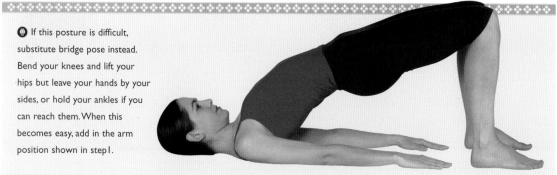

❹ If this posture is difficult, substitute bridge pose instead. Bend your knees and lift your hips but leave your hands by your sides, or hold your ankles if you can reach them. When this becomes easy, add in the arm position shown in step1.

salamba sarvangasana

SALAMBA = supported; SARVA = all or whole;

ANGA = limb or body; ASANA = posture

The rhythm of the practice changes with this pose, which is held for 25 breaths. This helps you wind down while maintaining heat and mental focus.

Exhale, lie in *Savasana* (see page 117) for a few breaths. Bring your palms flat to the floor and your legs together. Take a few breaths and roll up onto your shoulders with your hands on your back, elbows drawn in. Inhale, point your toes and lengthen your body. Stay for as long as you can, working up to 10, 15, 20 and 25 breaths. Go straight into the next pose: *Halasana*.

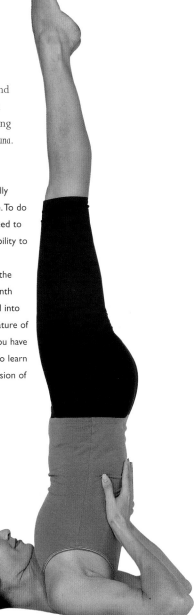

🔆 Shoulderstand is a potentially difficult and dangerous posture. To do it safely and beneficially, you need to develop enough shoulder flexibility to roll your shoulderblades right underneath your back so that the bony prominence of your seventh cervical vertebra is not pushed into the floor and the natural curvature of your neck is not flattened. If you have neck problems, it is advisable to learn this posture under the supervision of a good yoga teacher.

🌸 Nose

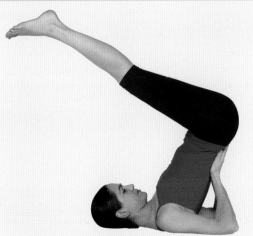

🌀 Although you can lessen the pressure on your neck in this pose by using blocks or blankets, one of the joys of Astanga yoga is its prop-free approach. So, if your neck feels uncomfortable, try dropping your hips much lower than vertical and supporting your hips or waist with your hands – this is a half-shoulderstand. Alternatively, lie flat on your back with your legs lifted straight up to the ceiling. This takes all the strain off your neck, but still gives you some of the benefits of inversion.

halasana

HALA = plough; ASANA = posture

This pose should be sharp and sturdy – keep your legs active throughout.

Maintain the focus on your breath and the *bandhas* as you ease into *Halasana*.

Exhale, slowly lower your feet to the floor over your head keeping your legs straight. Place your toes on the floor and keep lifting your hips upward, lengthening your spine. Take your hands off your back, interlace your fingers, straighten your arms and draw your hands down toward the floor behind you. Stay for five breaths and then go straight into the next pose: *Karnapidasana*.

🌸 Nose

🕉 *Halasana* gives your lower back muscles a deep stretch and, despite all the postures you have done in preparation, it can feel surprisingly strong. It is essential to go into *Halasana* slowly and carefully – don't collapse into the pose. Note that this posture differs from shoulderstand in that your weight is rolled a little further toward your head and off your shoulders. Curiously, this can feel easier than shoulderstand and so many people use *Halasana* as a preliminary pose, going first into *Halasana* for one breath, and then into shoulderstand.

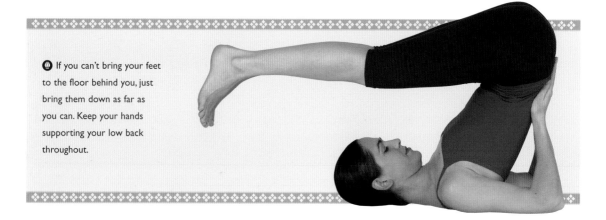

🌸 If you can't bring your feet to the floor behind you, just bring them down as far as you can. Keep your hands supporting your low back throughout.

karnapidasana

KARNA = ear; PIDA = pressure; ASANA = posture

Your focus becomes more inward with this pose. Listen to the rhythmic sound of your breath muffled by your knees closing in toward your ears.

Exhale, bend your knees and lower them to the floor either side of your head. Keep your arms in the same position as they were for *Halasana*. Gently press your knees toward your ears. Stay for five breaths and then go straight to the next pose: *Urdhva Padmasana*.

 Nose

🕉 Whether you find a pose easy or difficult often depends on the length and shape of your bones – not just how flexible or determined you are. For example, in this pose if you have a long back and shortish thighs, your knees have further to go to touch the floor and your neck will receive more pressure. So if you feel uncomfortable, don't strain. As always in yoga, go softly and slowly, feeling your way to the best expression of a posture.

❶ If you can't lower your knees without feeling uncomfortable pressure on your neck, just bend them and bring them in toward your forehead, still supporting your back with your hands.

urdhva padmasana

URDHVA = upward; PADMA = lotus; ASANA = posture

This perfectly poised balancing pose allows you to breathe with relative ease before you go on to the next variation in which the body is deeply folded.

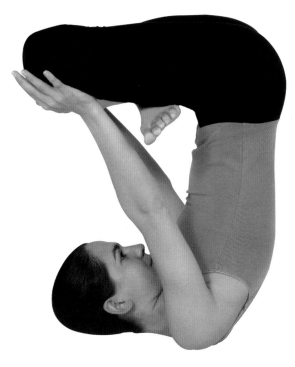

Inhale and lift your legs back up into a shoulderstand. Stabilize your body and find your balance. Exhale, fold your legs into the lotus position (see page 115) and place your hands under your knees with your arms straight to support the lotus. Stay for five breaths. Go straight into the next pose: *Pindasana*.

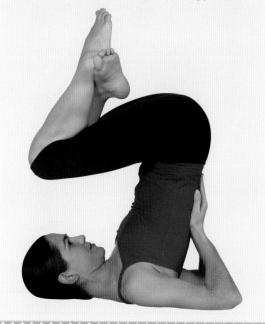

🌸 If you can't do the lotus position, then simply cross your ankles instead. Support your back with your hands as you cross your legs, then see if you can bring your hands to your knees. If not, keep your hands supporting your back.

🌸 Nose

🌀 As with *Karnapidasana*, this pose demands a supple neck. If you experience any kind of pain, modify or leave out the pose and substitute another shoulderstand. Your weight must be far enough back on your neck in order to balance the weight of your knees on your hands. This won't happen if your neck is stiff or you are worried about falling over backward. Concentrate on relaxing your knees onto your hands and letting your weight settle there. Your shoulders will almost prop the posture up. Use your abdominal muscles to help you to stay stable in the pose.

pindasana

PINDA = embryo; ASANA = posture

You can turn your awareness totally inward in this posture – it really does have something
of an embryonic feel. This is the last of the introverted poses – enjoy five quiet, still breaths.

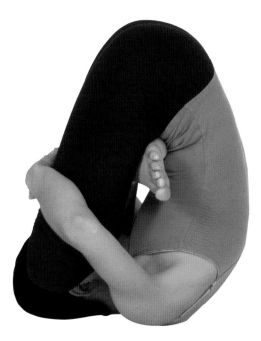

Exhale and lower your knees toward your chest and
wrap your arms around your legs, clasping your hands if
possible. Stay for five breaths. Go straight to the next pose:
Matsyasana.

✿ Nose

✸ Try to keep a little weight spreading through your shoulders
to maintain good support in this pose. The use of the *bandhas* will
help you to control your balance quite minutely. When you bring
your hands together in this pose, your weight tends to roll back.
If this creates undue pressure in your neck, roll out of the pose
straight away.

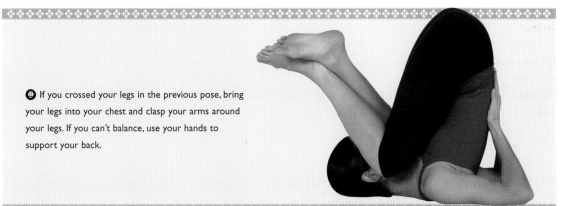

If you crossed your legs in the previous pose, bring
your legs into your chest and clasp your arms around
your legs. If you can't balance, use your hands to
support your back.

matsyasana

MATSYA = fish; ASANA = posture

It is said that one can float in water with the mouth and nose just lifted above the surface in this pose. The opening of the throat and chest has a celebratory feeling.

From *Pindasana* exhale, release your arms, bring your hands to the floor, palms down, and roll your spine slowly down out of *Pindasana* using the *bandhas* to help control your descent. Take hold of your feet with your hands and draw your elbows down toward the floor (but don't let them touch the floor). Lift your chest, expanding the front of your body and release your head back until the crown is resting on the floor. There should be very little weight on your head due to the up-thrust of your chest. Stay for five breaths. Go straight into the next pose: *Uttana Padasana*.

🌀 This is a long awaited backbend after the sequence of shoulderstands. Stay in it for more than five breaths if you need to.

🌸 Nose

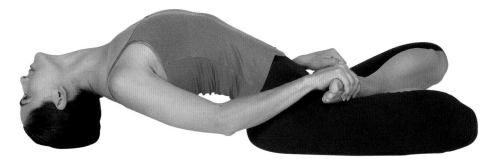

🌀 If your legs were crossed in *Pindasana*, keep them crossed and follow the instructions above. But rather than holding your feet, hold the tops of your thighs. Alternatively, do the pose by releasing your legs, stretching them out straight in front of you, placing your hands palms down underneath your buttocks, and pressing your elbows into the floor to help lift your chest. If this puts too much weight on your head or gives you discomfort in your neck, keep your head just off the floor.

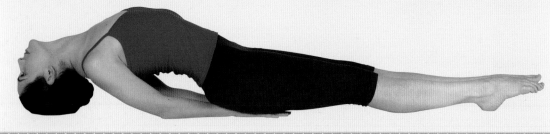

uttana padasana

UTTANA = extended; PADA = foot or leg; ASANA = posture

This is a fully extended variation of the previous pose. It has a similarly uplifting effect on the spirits.

❀ Nose

☯ Use the *bandhas* fully in order to protect your low back and energize the pose.

Inhale and stretch out your legs, lifting them 45 degrees off the floor with toes pointed and feet together. Keep the lift in your upper chest full and bring your palms together with your arms outstretched. Stay for five breaths. Go into a backward roll (see pages 98–99) and land in *Chaturanga* (see page 46). Inhale and go into up-facing dog. Exhale and go into down-facing dog. Come to a kneeling position for the next pose: *Sirsasana* A.

⚠ If it is too intense to hold your legs off the floor, lower them and just concentrate on raising your arms and the uplift of your chest.

sirsasana A

SIRSA = head; ASANA = posture

Known as the "king" of yoga postures, the headstand is placed almost at the very end of the practice. This position in the sequence suggests that poise and equilibrium are required rather than huge effort.

✿ Nose

⊙ If you can't get into a full headstand, practice the preliminary steps until you gain confidence. If you find it hard to get your feet off the floor, try lifting your legs with your knees bent – this takes less abdominal strength. Keep practising the straight leg version every now and then so that eventually you can do it with ease. It is better for your balance and confidence to practice in the centre of a room rather than against a wall.

Kneel down and place your elbows shoulder-width apart on the floor (you can measure this by holding your elbows with your hands). Clasp your hands, letting your lower little finger slip into the inside of your palm, so that the sides of both hands rest easily on the floor. Exhale, gently place the back of your head into your palms with the crown of your head resting on the floor. Inhale, straighten your legs and walk your feet toward your head as far as you can, while maintaining broad shoulders and a long neck. Now tilt your hips backward over your head so that you can bring your feet off the floor slowly, keeping your legs straight. Lift your legs to vertical. Softly ground your head and elbows without strain. Balance. Stay for 25 breaths or as long as you can without discomfort. Go straight into the next pose: *Sirsasana B*.

sirsasana B

Exhale and lower your legs down to a horizontal position. You need to push your hips back beyond your head to provide a counterbalance to your legs – it may take a little time to get the hang of this. Make the pose strong by fully utilizing the abdominal control of the *bandhas*. Stay for five breaths. Inhale, go back into a full headstand. Exhale, lower your feet to the floor. Remain with your head down for a few moments before going into a vinyasa.

🌓 Nose

🌑 If you can't find the strength to balance with your legs horizontal, bend your knees toward your chest as you lower your legs. Stay for five breaths and then return to a headstand. Aim to work toward slowly letting your legs straighten. Above all, try to hold the pose steady.

baddha padmasana

BADDHA = bound; PADMA = lotus; ASANA = posture

The series draws to a close with three poses based on the lotus position. Lotus flowers are symbolic of peace and inner harmony. The binding in this pose adds a sense of stability and grounding.

Exhale, bring your legs into lotus position by placing your right foot on your left thigh and your left foot on your right thigh. Both feet should be as close as possible to your hip sockets. Take your left hand behind your back to hold your left foot and then reach your right hand around your back to hold your right foot. Inhale, lengthen your spine. Stay for five breaths. Exhale, fold forward bringing your head toward the floor. Stay for five breaths. Inhale, release your hands and place them on the floor just behind your hips about shoulder-width apart. Roll your chest up and open, and let your head tilt back. Take five breaths. Go straight to the next pose: *Padmasana*.

✤ Third eye

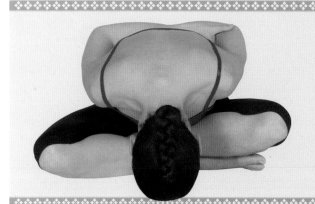

🔵 If you can't do a full lotus position, do half-lotus or cross your legs instead. Then cross your arms behind your back and hold your elbows. Fold forward in this position.

padmasana

PADMA = lotus; ASANA = posture

The 10 breaths in simple lotus position prepare you for the following and final challenge of the Primary Series.

Exhale, bring your hands to your knees, palms facing upward, and make the seal of consciousness – *chin mudra* – by bringing your index finger and thumb together. Sit upright and bring your chin down toward your throat to make *jalandhara bandha*, the throat lock. Stay for 10 breaths. Go straight into the next posture: *Tolasana*.

🕉 Focus on the quality of your breath and the gentle up-lifting of your spine.

🌼 Nose

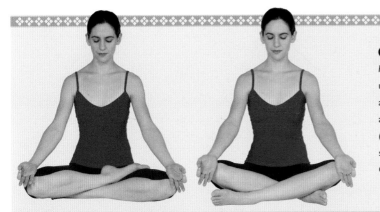

⚫ The most important thing about *Padmasana* is that you are able to sit upright with a long spine and breathe softly and smoothly. If your knees or ankles hurt, abandon the pose and get into half-lotus (far left) or half-adepts pose, in which you simply cross one heel in front of the other. Or you can just cross your legs (left).

tolasana

TOLA = scales; ASANA = posture ·

This is the final ascent! Hopefully you will be able to employ a mind over matter strength summoned from deep *within* to complete the challenge of *Tolasana*.

Exhale, bring your hands to the floor beside your hips. Inhale, press your hands into the floor, lift your knees toward your chest and bring your whole body off the floor to balance like a weighing scale. Stay for 25 slow breaths before going into a vinyasa.

❀ Nose

☯ Whether you are doing the full pose or the modification, a full *mula bandha* will help you to keep your legs lifted. This posture is sometimes held for 100 deep, fast breaths rather than 25 slow ones – the choice is yours!

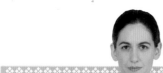

🌀 If you can't do a lotus position comfortably, get into a crossed-leg position, lift your legs up and hold onto your feet. You can also try pressing down on the floor with your hands to lift yourself up. This presents more of a challenge – if you can't hold the pose for 25 breaths, just do as much as you can without strain.

savasana

SAVA = corpse; ASANA = posture

The simple stillness of this pose holds an astounding depth after the constant flow and energy of the Primary Series: deep peace, deep stillness, deep rest. Cover yourself with a blanket as your body temperature will drop as you rest.

Exhale, lie down on your back with your feet a little way apart and your palms facing up, about 20–30cm (8–12ins) from your sides. Relax your body completely. Stop using the *ujjayi* breathing technique (see page 36) and, instead, breathe a soft, easy breath. Rest. Stay in this position at least until your breathing and heartbeat return to their normal resting rate and, if you can, stay for 15 minutes or longer. Don't fall asleep – your aim is to reach a state of deep, conscious relaxation.

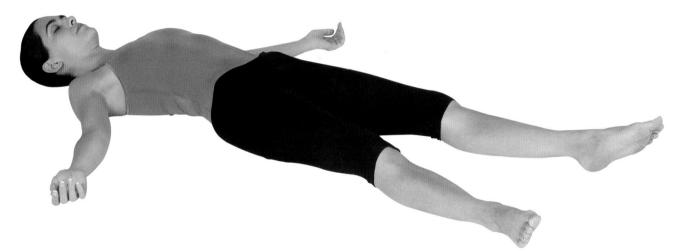

⚛ The Primary Series is like an enormous meal that you must leave time to digest. And *Savasana* gives you the opportunity to do this. Although it is a posture of physical rest, it needs to be approached with the same care and attention as all the others in the sequence (don't be tempted to think of *Tolasana* as the final pose). *Savasana* allows you to assimilate all that has gone before on a physical, mental, emotional, energetic and spiritual level. Take your time to absorb the effects of the practice and let yourself come full circle with this wonderful, deep and well-deserved rest. Most importantly, don't rush through *Savasana* so that you can get going with your next task.

adapted practice
for beginners

This short, adapted sequence contains just 10 postures from the Primary Series, in the order in which they appear in the full sequence. There is a balanced sample of standing, seated, forward-bending, back-bending, twisting and inverted poses that are useful to practise on days when you don't have time to go to a class but would like to do some self-practice. This sequence is also good if you are relatively new to Astanga yoga. Start by doing sun salutation A five times.

SUN SALUTATION A (SEE PAGES 46–47)

ADAPTED PRACTICE FOR BEGINNERS

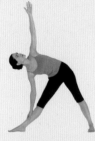
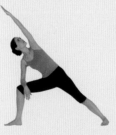
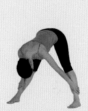
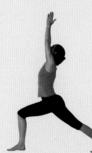
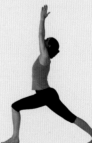
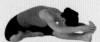
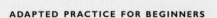

Utthita Trikonasana
(see page 56)

Utthita Parsvakonasana
(see page 58)

Prasarita
Padottanasana A
(see page 60)

Virabhadrasana A
(see page 68)

Janu Sirsasana A
(see page 79)

The traditional way to learn Astanga yoga is to start by learning the sun salutations (see pages 46–53), and then mastering one posture of the Primary Series at a time. This produces a steady learning curve and curbs the tendency to push yourself beyond your limits.

Marichyasana C
(see page 84)

Navasana
(see page 86)

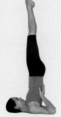

Salamba
Sarvangasana
(see page 105)

Matsyasana
(see page 110)

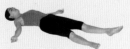

Savasana
(see page 117)

a short practice for all

The entire Primary Series takes a real expert about 90 minutes to complete. It takes me nearer two hours and at first you may struggle to get it done in less than that. If you don't have much time but you would like to get a taste of the Primary Series, the following practice should take you around an hour to complete. All the postures are taken from the Primary Series in the order in which they normally appear. Start by doing sun salutations A and B (see pages 46–53) five times each.

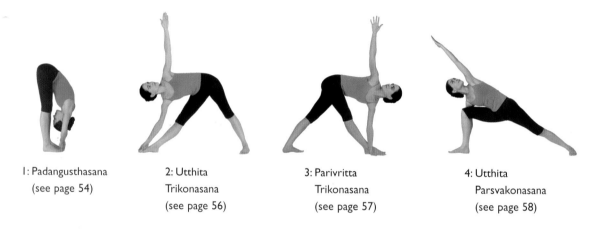

1: Padangusthasana
(see page 54)

2: Utthita
Trikonasana
(see page 56)

3: Parivritta
Trikonasana
(see page 57)

4: Utthita
Parsvakonasana
(see page 58)

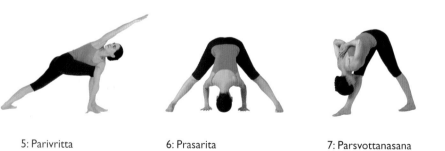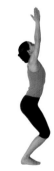

5: Parivritta
Parsvakonasana
(see page 59)

6: Prasarita
Padottanasana A
(see page 60)

7: Parsvottanasana
(see page 62)

8: Utkatasana
(see page 67)

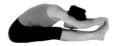

9: Paschimottanasana A
(see page 75)

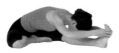

10: Janu Sirsasana A
(see page 79)

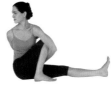

11: Marichyasana C
(see page 84)

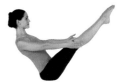

12: Navasana
(see page 86)

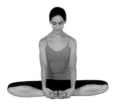

13: Baddha
Konasana A
(see page 92)

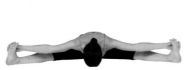

14: Upavishta
Konasana A
(see page 94)

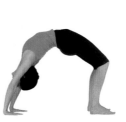

15: Urdhva
Dhanurasana
(see page 104)

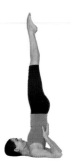

16: Salamba
sarvangasana
(see page 105)

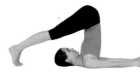

17: Halasana
(see page 106)

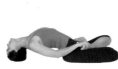

18: Matsyasana
(see page 110)

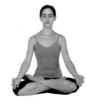

19: Padmasana
(see page 115)

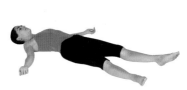

20: Savasana
(see page 117)

sun salutations

SUN SALUTATION A

🕉 The vinyasa, or order of movements in any sequence is ascribed a number. Traditionally these numbers are called out by a teacher as a shorthand for the long Sanskrit names. Below are the Sanskrit numbers for the vinyasa of the sun salutations.

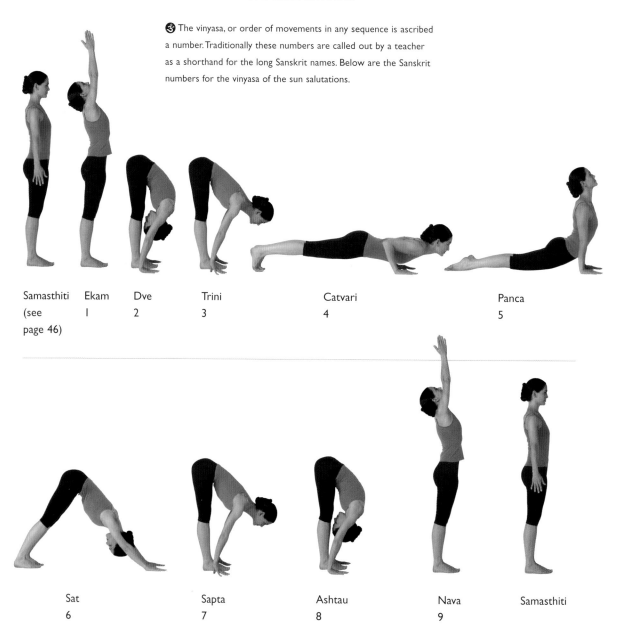

Samasthiti
(see
page 46)

Ekam
1

Dve
2

Trini
3

Catvari
4

Panca
5

Sat
6

Sapta
7

Ashtau
8

Nava
9

Samasthiti

SUN SALUTATION B

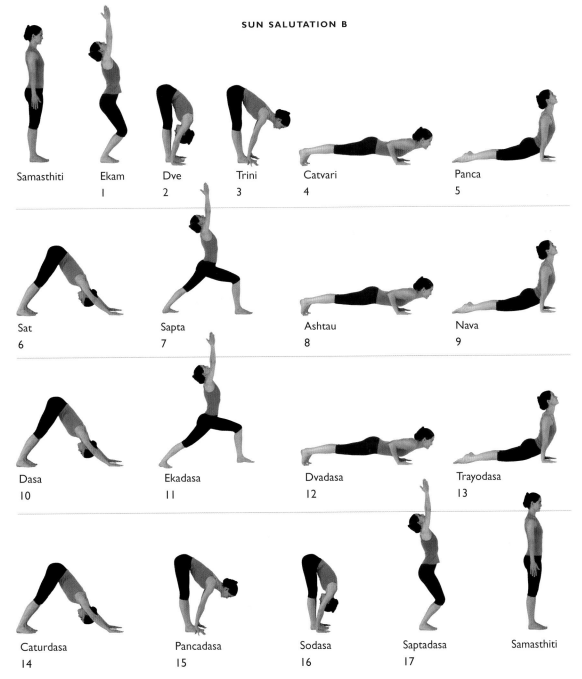

Samasthiti

Ekam
1

Dve
2

Trini
3

Catvari
4

Panca
5

Sat
6

Sapta
7

Ashtau
8

Nava
9

Dasa
10

Ekadasa
11

Dvadasa
12

Trayodasa
13

Caturdasa
14

Pancadasa
15

Sodasa
16

Saptadasa
17

Samasthiti

standing poses

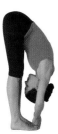

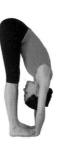

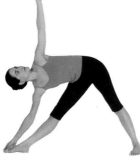

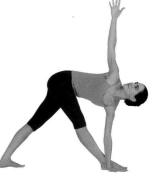

1: Padangusthasana
(see page 54)

2: Padahastasana
(see page 55)

3: Utthita Trikonasana
(see page 56)

4: Parivritta Trikonasana
(see page 57)

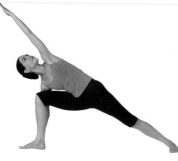

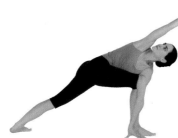

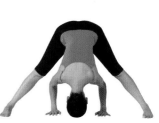

5: Utthita Parsvakonasana
(see page 58)

6: Parivritta Parsvakonasana
(see page 59)

7: Prasarita Padottanasana A
(see page 60)

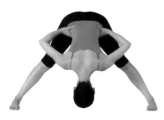

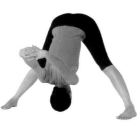

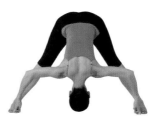

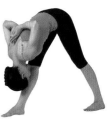

8: Prasarita Padottanasana B
(see page 61)

9: Prasarita Padottanasana C
(see page 61)

10: Prasarita Padottanasana D
(see page 61)

11: Parsvottanasana
(see page 62)

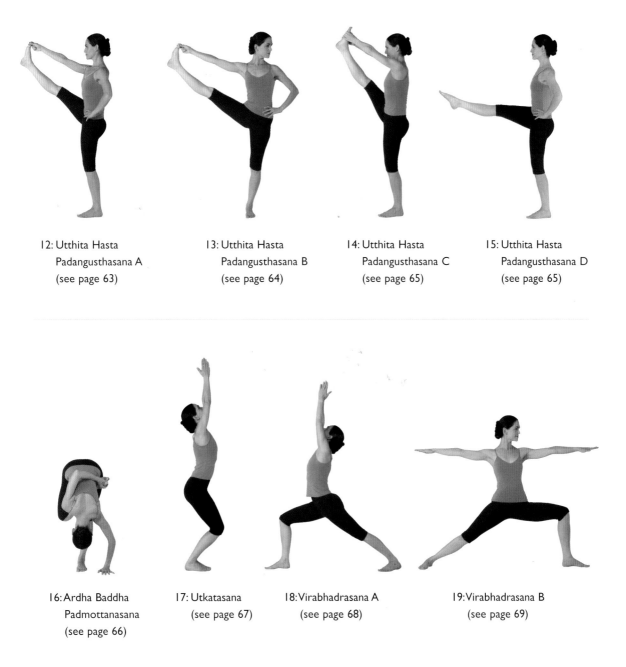

12: Utthita Hasta
    Padangusthasana A
    (see page 63)

13: Utthita Hasta
    Padangusthasana B
    (see page 64)

14: Utthita Hasta
    Padangusthasana C
    (see page 65)

15: Utthita Hasta
    Padangusthasana D
    (see page 65)

16: Ardha Baddha
    Padmottanasana
    (see page 66)

17: Utkatasana
    (see page 67)

18: Virabhadrasana A
    (see page 68)

19: Virabhadrasana B
    (see page 69)

seated poses

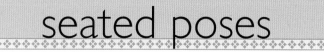

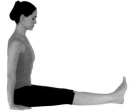

1: Dandasana (see page 74)

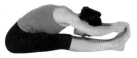

2: Paschimottanasana A
(see page 75)

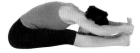

3: Paschimottanasana B
(see page 75)

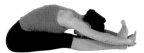

4: Paschimottanasana C
(see page 75)

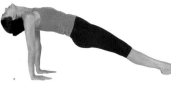

5: Purvottanasana
(see page 76)

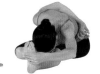

6: Ardha Baddha
Padma
Paschimottanasana
(see page 77)

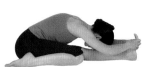

7: Trianga Mukhaikapada
Paschimottanasana
(see page 78)

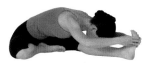

8: Janu Sirsasana A
(see page 79)

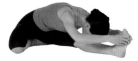

9: Janu Sirsasana B
(see page 80)

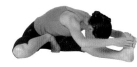

10: Janu Sirsasana C
(see page 81)

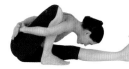

11: Marichyasana A
(see page 82)

12: Marichyasana B
(see page 83)

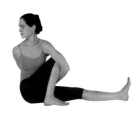

13: Marichyasana C
(see page 84)

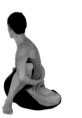

14: Marichyasana D
(see page 85)

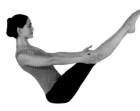

15: Navasana
(see page 86)

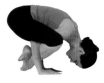

16: Bhujapidasana
(see page 87)

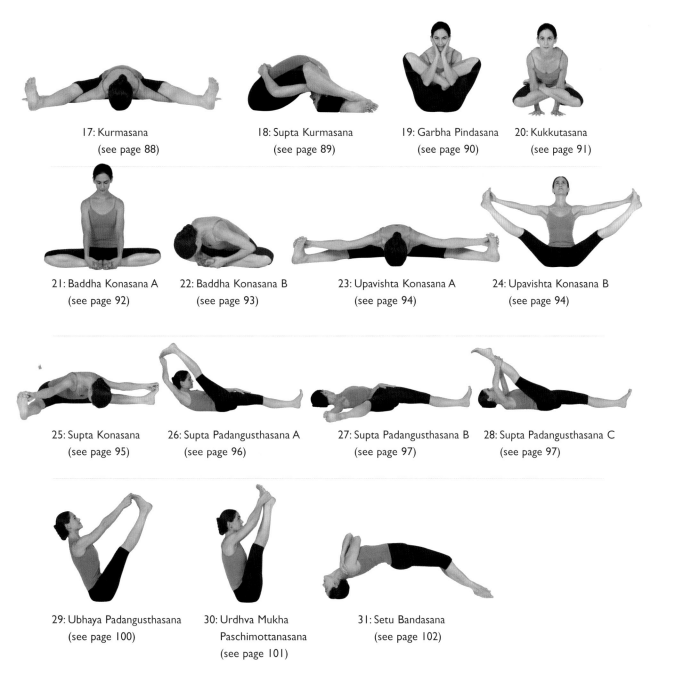

17: Kurmasana
(see page 88)

18: Supta Kurmasana
(see page 89)

19: Garbha Pindasana
(see page 90)

20: Kukkutasana
(see page 91)

21: Baddha Konasana A
(see page 92)

22: Baddha Konasana B
(see page 93)

23: Upavishta Konasana A
(see page 94)

24: Upavishta Konasana B
(see page 94)

25: Supta Konasana
(see page 95)

26: Supta Padangusthasana A
(see page 96)

27: Supta Padangusthasana B
(see page 97)

28: Supta Padangusthasana C
(see page 97)

29: Ubhaya Padangusthasana
(see page 100)

30: Urdhva Mukha
Paschimottanasana
(see page 101)

31: Setu Bandasana
(see page 102)

finishing sequence

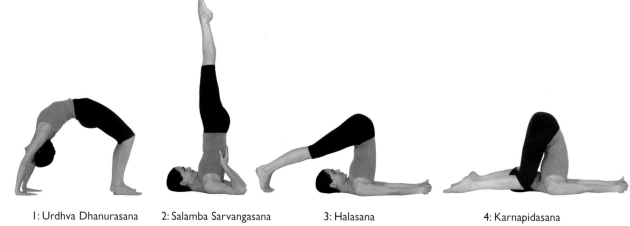
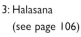

1: Urdhva Dhanurasana
(see page 104)

2: Salamba Sarvangasana
(see page 105)

3: Halasana
(see page 106)

4: Karnapidasana
(see page 107)

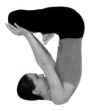
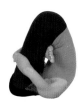
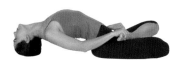

5: Urdhva Padmasana
(see page 108)

6: Pindasana
(see page 109)

7: Matsyasana
(see page 110)

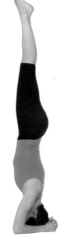
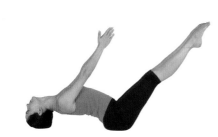
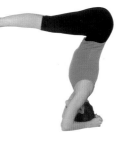

8: Uttana Padasana
(see page 111)

9: Sirsasana A
(see page 112)

10: Sirsasana B
(see page 113)

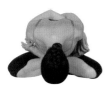
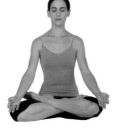
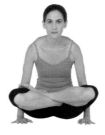
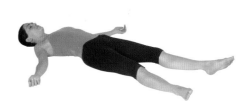

11: Baddha Padmasana
(see page 114)

12: Padmasana
(see page 115)

13: Tolasana
(see page 116)

14: Savasana
(see page 117)

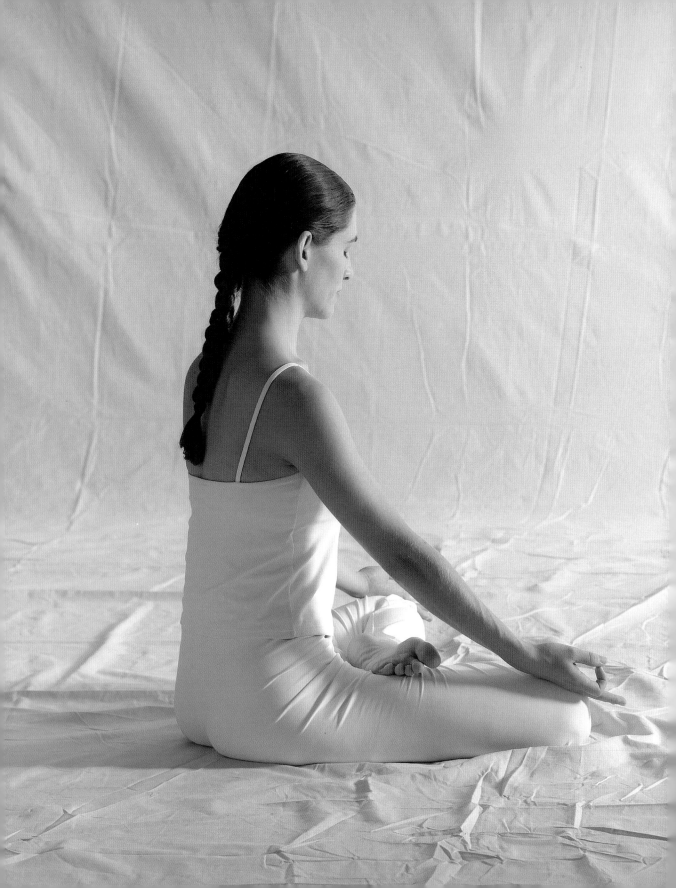

chapter five

further study

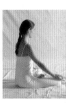

Once started, yoga can become a lifelong practice. Whatever stage you are at there is always something more to learn and a way to go deeper. In this chapter I look at the traditional relationships between teachers and their students, and the idea of self-practice as a route to development. There are suggestions of ways to deepen or broaden an already well established practice, and a list of helpful addresses and organizations to refer to for more assistance. Yoga communities all over the world are supportive and generous to those who seek knowledge in good faith. Among them the Astanga yoga community stand out as the most astonishingly well-connected and closely knit. They make full use of modern technology with a great deal of information being shared on websites and through email, and you will be welcomed at practice sessions worldwide by people who share your interest in this unique form of self-development.

finding a teacher

If you have not practised Astanga yoga before, you will need to learn from a teacher. An experienced teacher can not only help you to do the postures correctly, but can also help you to temper your practice to make it fine and delicate, as well as introspective, reflective, meditative and nourishing. Without these refinements you risk not just injury to your muscles or joints, but also developing a practice that is hollow, "external" and, ultimately, boring!

Teacher training in Astanga yoga

The traditional way of learning yoga in India is by studying with a guru (teacher), often for a considerable number of years. At a certain point the teacher deems the student experienced enough to undertake students of their own. This system is known as the *guru parampara*, which literally means "one after another". The modern guru of Astanga yoga, Shri K Pattabhi Jois, has "certificated" a very small number of students to teach Astanga yoga in the West – this means that he has assessed their practice and given them his blessing to pass on the Astanga yoga tradition to their own students.

However, because of the sudden and massive popularity of Astanga yoga in the West, there aren't enough certificated teachers to meet the demand. The system for training yoga teachers in the West is almost entirely unregulated, and there is no official body for the training of Astanga yoga teachers – many of whom are fiercely loyal to their guru and would not consider a teacher training course with anyone else.

Although no organization exists for training teachers specifically in Astanga yoga there are organizations for training teachers in Hatha yoga (see page 12). In the UK this organization is the British Wheel of Yoga (BWY). A long-term practitioner of Astanga yoga who also has a BWY qualification will have a good understanding of yoga in its widest context, anatomy and physiology, and the relationship between yoga and health.

What to look for

Because Astanga yoga lacks a formal system of qualifications, you may need to rely on your own personal judgement and instinct when choosing a teacher. Look for someone you respect and trust. A good teacher takes your yoga practice seriously and has a solid and stable background of practice and teaching themselves. Word of mouth is often a good way to find a teacher.

Beware of teachers who have a reputation for being extreme or outrageous in their teaching – Astanga yoga is not performance art! Also, bear in mind that an impressive looking personal practice is not necessarily evidence of a good teaching technique.

Once you find a teacher you like, stick with them for as long as possible. Consistency in the way that you are taught has a very beneficial effect on your understanding of yoga, especially if you are a beginner.

What happens in a class

Your teacher will guide you through the movements of the Primary Series using a combination of demonstration, verbal instruction and correction. A good teacher will go slowly enough for you to grasp the basics of each posture as you go along. In many Astanga yoga classes teachers want to maintain the flow and heat of the practice, so they will not stop for detailed explanations and corrections. This may be a bit disquieting if you have previously studied a different style of yoga and are not accustomed to such speed – but it can be beneficial to flow through the movements without over-analyzing them. This way, you stay in your body and not in your head!

Your teacher will probably use physical adjustments. These may take the form of gentle pressure to help you dis-

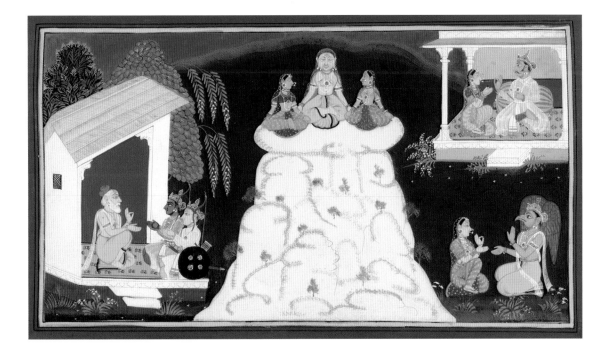

cover a better alignment in a posture or they may be very deep and strong movements in which your teacher pushes or presses their body weight against you to help you move deeper into a posture. You will also get help and support learning some of the more complicated poses in the Primary Series, such as dropping backward into *Urdhva Dhanurasana* (see page 104), crossing your legs behind your head in *Supta Kurmasana* (see page 89) or getting into headstand poses (see *Sirsasana A* on page 112).

Performed well, adjustments are marvellous learning experiences that can feel exhilarating. However, done badly or inappropriately, they can cause you discomfort and pain. If any adjustment feels too strong or you just don't like the way it feels, say so – never allow a teacher to inflict pain. All teachers need feedback from their students in order that they can learn themselves. A good teacher will never be offended by feedback.

In this scene from the *Ramayana* – one of India's greatest epic tales – King Sagara (at the top of the mound in the middle) is shown practising yoga accompanied by his consorts in order to gain a boon and be granted a child.

Studying in India

A trip to the Astanga Yoga Research Institute in Mysore to be taught by Shri K Pattabhi Jois or his grandson Sharath, has become a necessary pilgrimage for serious students of Astanga yoga. Since the new yoga *shala* (school) has been built, prices have risen to almost Western standards and the pressure for places is as high as ever. If you are able to go, try to allow a reasonably lengthy visit. To discover what a visit to Mysore entails, talk to someone from your local Astanga class or look at websites on which people have posted their "Mysore experiences". Both Shri K Pattabhi Jois and Sharath also regularly teach abroad. For details about visiting Mysore or international tours, see page 138.

self-practice

Once you have learned at least the sun salutations (see pages 46–53) and are familiar with the basics of *ujjayi* breathing and the *bandhas*, you can practise Astanga yoga by youself. You can either attend a self-practice class with a teacher on hand for guidance – these classes are sometimes known as Mysore-style classes – or you can practise at home on your own.

Some of the main advantages of self-practice are that you get to know the sequence of postures intimately, and over time you develop a high level of self-discipline and self-observation. Self-practice is particularly useful if you are unable to attend regular yoga classes – if you travel a lot, for example. The only things you need to practise by yourself are a small amount of space, a yoga mat and time.

Mysore-style classes

In Mysore-style or self-practice classes (Mysore is the home of Shri K Pattabhi Jois' Astanga Yoga Research Institute; see page 138), students practise the postures at their own pace. Classes may last for three hours or more. This doesn't mean that you have to arrive at the beginning of a class and practise for a full three hours – instead you can come and do as much as you want, and go when you have finished your own practice, even if everyone else is still doing theirs. Everyone is likely to be doing different postures at different times. Some students may be relative beginners, and others may be doing the Second or even Third Series.

At Mysore-style classes the role of the teacher is to help you by offering corrections and adjustments when you need them and, leaving you to get on with your practice when you don't. This is one of the most wonderful aspects of this type of class; you are able to practise in a group but, instead of feeling that you have to keep up with others, you can go at your own pace. You have access to a teacher's watchful eye and helping hands, but in a less intense atmosphere than a one-to-one session. You can develop self-reliance and self-observation in *asana* practice without the risk of repeating mistakes because you are not aware of them.

Practising at home

Many people attend a taught class for years and, despite the fact that they are repeating the same sequence over and over again, they are unable to recall the order of postures by themselves. If you only ever practice in a taught class there is always a little bit of your mind that is not completely focused on the task in hand.

This is why it is good to do self-practice without a teacher as often as you can. Although self-practice feels very

STARTING SELF-PRACTICE

If you have never practised yoga by yourself, here are some ideas that will help you to get started and sustain your practice over time.

- Practise in a peaceful environment. Minimize distractions.
- Don't be over ambitious at the beginning – a few rounds of sun salutation are fine to start off with. Add more postures when you feel ready.
- Go slowly and methodically. Self-practice is the perfect opportunity to pay proper attention to your own breathing without the distraction of other people around you.
- Always close a practice with the finishing sequence or a modification of it. Don't rush to do something else – relax for a few minutes and observe the effects of your practice.

different to doing yoga in a taught class, it is worth developing because, ultimately, self-reliance makes your practice genuinely yours and, over time, you will be rewarded with a stronger, more autonomous yoga practice.

Many people, especially those just starting Astanga yoga, find the prospect of self-practice a daunting one. Motivating yourself to practise alone can be difficult, and students worry that they will make mistakes that will go uncorrected. The best way to start is to practise only those postures about which you feel confident. For example, you don't need to do the whole of the Primary Series; try doing a few rounds of sun salutations instead.

As for making mistakes, that is one of the best ways of learning! If you are mindful and steady in your practice, you will know if something is badly wrong because it will hurt. The Primary Series is very challenging – physically and mentally – and quite impossible to get perfect (if there is such a thing) first time round. It needs years of consistent practise to develop an accomplished form. Yoga is about the journey, not the goal – enjoy the scenery as you pass by. Feeling frustrated at the limitations of the physical body is one of Astanga yoga's hardest mental challenges, and one that we all face sooner or later. There is an old proverb: "The woods would be very silent if no birds sang but the best."

Regular self-practice is the best way to build up a intimate knowledge of the Primary Series. As Shri K Pattabhi Jois is fond of saying: "Practice, practice; all is coming."

ways to go deeper

As your Astanga yoga practice becomes established, you may want to learn more about yoga in general or to examine your own practice in further detail. There are many facets of the practice to explore from a detailed physical exploration of each pose in the series to meditation. Reading and studying are also routes to a deeper understanding of yoga (these can be useful especially if you have temporary or permanent physical limitations). The possibilities are endless – here are a few ideas to start you off.

Physical exploration

If you would like a deeper understanding of the physical aspects of each pose in the Primary Series, there are many specialist worshops that you can attend. Some concentrate on the anatomy and physiology of yoga, others relate to theoretical and philosophical ideas, such as the *chakra* system. Many well-known teachers regularly hold workshops to help students develop a particular aspect of their practice, for example, how to "jump through" or improve your headstand.

You may find that going to classes in a different style of yoga also helps to inform your Astanga practice. Iyengar yoga teachers in particular have an astounding wealth of knowledge on the anatomical precision of yoga *asana* and can help you to refine your postures and clarify your practice.

Pranayama is a good next step once you have grasped the basics of *asana* practice. Some teachers specialize in teaching these breathing techniques. Originally, Shri K Pattabhi Jois taught them to his students along with the *asana*, but he seems to do this less often today. You may need to look to a different school of yoga to find a really experienced *pranayama* teacher – but it is well worth it.

One way of deepening your understanding of Astanga yoga is to devote each practice session to a specific aspect of yoga, such as your breath.

Meditation

You need a great deal of concentration to complete the Primary Series, and you can tap into and utilize this when you start a meditation practice. Begin by trying to keep your mind at a quiet and focused point at the end of each *asana* practice. Try to stay in this meditative state for a little longer each time. Over time you may discover that you can get into this mind state without practising the entire Primary Series first. It may be beneficial to try a quiet seated meditation that is independent of your *asana* practice, for example, at night.

Reading and studying

There is a great deal of inspirational literature connected with yoga, ranging from the poetic and mystical to the practical and prosaic. Many yoga practitioners have written about how yoga has helped them through difficult times in their lives. There are diaries by total novices and world experts making the trip to see *Guruji* (see pages 14–15) for the first or the 15th time, and there are many excellent technical manuals available (see page 139).

You can also study the ancient yoga texts. It makes sense to start with the classical *Yoga Sutras* and the eight limbs of yoga described by Patanjali (see pages 18–19). Ask yourself whether you can integrate these ideals into your yoga practice and your life in general. The *Yama* and *Niyama* (social and individual conduct respectively) provide a relatively simple set of instructions about how to live. But when you consider each one, you may find some more palatable than others! Can you maintain a dedication to what you are practising, and an open mind and friendly attitude? Have you become overbearing, pompous or moralizing toward others since discovering the wonders of Astanga yoga? If so, think again!

The *Yoga Sutras* are best studied with a teacher in the traditional way. This study explores the potential of the human mind. You may be able to find a beginners' course that lasts just a few days. If you wish to continue, the ideal way of studying the *Yoga Sutras* in detail is one-to-one with a teacher.

There are many excellent modern books on Ayurveda (the traditional Indian system of medicine that uses yoga as both a preventive and curative tool). Gaining an insight into your Ayurvedic constitution (see pages 28–29) can provide useful dietary and lifestyle guidelines, and help you balance your life to get the most out of your yoga practice. If you become interested in Ayurveda, a personal consultation with an Ayurvedic doctor will provide you with an accurate constitutional analysis.

EXPLORING A POSE

During your self-practice (see pages 134–135), try giving each one of your practice sessions a distinct focus. Here are some ideas:

- Concentrate on the positioning of your hands and feet and how they support you in a pose. Bring your awareness to the inner and outer edges of your feet and the grounding of your big toes and index fingers, especially in down-facing dog (see page 47). Observe how you spring, land and roll over on your feet.

- Focus on keeping your shoulders and upper chest wide and soft. Throughout your practice, remember to inhale fully and expand your upper body. Be aware of the movement of your shoulderblades, both in postures where your arms are supporting your body and in postures where your arms are free.

- Do a full practice prioritizing your breath over everything else at all times. Modify the poses if you need to so that you can keep your breath totally smooth and regular.

astanga yoga organizations

In the UK

John Scott

www.johnscottashtanga.co.uk

The Yoga Studio

The Old Newlyn School

3-4 Off Kenstella Road

Newlyn

Penzance

TR18 5AB

In the US

Richard Freeman

The Yoga Workshop

2020 21st Street

Boulder

CO 80302

Eddie and Jocelyn Stern

Patanjali Yoga Shala

611 Broadway Suite 203

New York

NY 10012

David Swenson

www.ashtanga.net

In Australia

Dena Kingsberg

PO Box 1443

Byron Bay

NSW 2481

Graeme Northfield

PO Box 220

Cooroy

Queensland 4563

In India

Shri K Pattabhi Jois

Astanga Yoga Nilayam

876/1 1st cross

Laxmipuram

Mysore 570004

In Italy

Lino Miele

Via Cassia 698

00189 Rome

Italy

www.astanga.it

bibliography and videos/DVDs

Books

Bernard, Theos *Hatha Yoga* (Essence of Health Publishing, South Africa, 2001)

Bihar School of Yoga *Hatha Yoga Pradipika* (Bihar School of Yoga, Munger, India, 1985)

Bouanchaud, Bernard *The Essence of Yoga – Reflections on the Yoga Sutras of Patanjali* (Rudra Press, Portland, Oregon, 1997)

Buddhananda, Swami *Moola Bandha – The Master Key* (Bihar School of Yoga, Munger, India, 1996)

Coulter, David *Anatomy of Hatha Yoga* (Body and Breath, Honesdale, Pennsylvania, 2001)

De Michelis, Elizabeth *A History of Modern Yoga* (Continuum, London and New York, 2004)

Desikachar, TKV *Reflections on Yoga Sutra of Patanjali* (includes chanting CD) (Krishnamacharya Yoga Mandiram, Chennai, India, 2003)

Desikachar, TKV and Desikachar, Kausthub *Adi Sankara's Yoga Taravali* (Krishnamacharya Yoga Mandiram, Chennai, India, 2003)

Desikachar, TKV and Ravens, RH *Health, Healing and Beyond* (Aperture, New York, 1998)

Desikachar, TKV *The Heart of Yoga* (Inner Traditions International, Rochester, Vermont, 1995)

Fraser, Tara *Yoga for You* (Duncan Baird Publishers, London 2001/Thorsons, New York, 2001)

Feuerstein, G *The Yoga Tradition* (Hohm Press, Prescott, Arizona, 1998)

Frawley, David *Yoga and Ayurveda* (Lotus Press, Twin Lakes, Wisconsin, 1999)

Freedman, Françoise Babira *Yoga for Pregnancy, Birth and Beyond* (Dorling Kindersley, London and New York, 2004)

Freedman, Françoise Babira and Hall, Doriel *Postnatal Yoga* (Lorenz Books, London, 2000)

Iyengar, BKS *Light on the Yoga Sutras of Patanjali* (Thorsons, London and New York, 1996)

Iyengar, BKS *Light on Yoga* (Thorsons, London, 1991/Schocken, New York, 1995)

Jois, Shri K Pattabhi *Yoga Mala* (Eddie Stern, New York, 1999)

Miele, Lino *Astanga Yoga* (Lino Miele, Rome, 1996)

Rosen, Richard *The Yoga of Breath* (Shambhala Publications, Boston, 2002)

Scott, John *Astanga Yoga* (Gaia Books, London, 2002/Three Rivers Press, New York, 2004)

Singleton, Mark *Yoga for You and Your Child* (Duncan Baird Publishers, London 2004/Thorsons, New York, 2004)

Sjoman, NE *The Yoga Tradition of the Mysore Palace* (Abhinav Publications, New Delhi, 1996)

Stern, Eddie and Summerbell, Deirdre *Shri K Pattabhi Jois: A Tribute* (Eddie Stern and Gwyneth Paltrow, New York, 2002)

David Swenson *Astanga Yoga – The Practice Manual* (Astanga Yoga Productions, Austin, Texas, 1999)

Teasdill, Wendy *Yoga for Pregnancy* (Gaia Books, London, 1999)

Videos and DVDs

Good videos and DVDs of the Astanga Yoga system are available by the following teachers:
Richard Freeman
John Scott
David Swenson

index

acknowledgments

Picture credits

The publisher would like to thank
the following people, museums and
photographic libraries for permission
to reproduce their material. Every care
has been taken to trace copyright
holders. However, if we have omitted
anyone, we apologise and will, if
informed, make corrections in any
future edition.

page 12 Corbis/Liba Taylor; page 13
KYM Archives; page 15 Dinodia Photo
Library, Mumbai/T S Satyan; page
16 Dinodia Photo Library, Mumbai;
page 19 AKG-images/British Library;
page 20 Dinodia Photo Library,
Mumbai/T S Satyan; page 25
Corbis/Dennis Degnan, page 30
Corbis/Raoul Minsart; page 34 Art
Archive, London/Musée Guimet/Dagli
Orti; page 133 British Library, London.

Model

Tara Fraser

Consultant at photographic shoots

Nigel Jones

Make-up artists

Jo Jenkins
Fay De Bremaeker
Tinks Reding

Author's acknowledgments

I am enormously grateful to the many
people who have generously lent
their time, energy and talents to this
project, either directly or indirectly.
My special thanks to Nigel Jones,
Matthew Ward, Mark Singleton,
Dr Elizabeth de Michelis (DHIIR,
University of Cambridge), Dagmar
Benner, Kesta Desmond, Dan Sturges,
Julia Charles, Alison Batley and
Autumn Jacobsen.

Tara Fraser can be contacted at:
Yoga Junction,
Unit 24 City North,
Fonthill Road, Finsbury Park,
London N4 3HF
020 7263 3113
info@yogajunction.co.uk
www.yogajunction.co.uk